LOW CHOLESTEROL FOOD LIST

BOOST GOOD HDL CHOLESTEROL FOODS TO EAT, LOWER BAD LDL CHOLESTEROL WITH FOODS TO AVOID, 40 TASTY LOW-CHOLESTEROL RECIPES, 30 DAY MEAL PLAN, A QUICK REFERENCE POCKET GUIDE

JULIA MEADOWS

ABOUT THE AUTHOR

Julia Meadows is a health professional and wellness expert, specialising in nutrition she has delivered life-changing transformations for her readers.

She's residing with her family; husband, 2 boys and a girl, 2 cats and dog in the beautiful countryside of Sussex, just outside of London, England.

As a master health & wellness expert Julia teaches clients on consciousness, mindful living, nutrition, health care and diet, and good food for the mind, body and soul. Through our teaching Julia has helped clients worldwide gain a better advantage and help develop themselves and achieve more from what they desire.

She's in the changing lives business.

TAKE YOUR LIFESTYLE JOURNEY TO THE NEXT LEVEL!

http://www.facebook.com/groups/glycemic/

In our exclusive Diabetic and Low-Glycemic Information group, you'll connect with like-minded individuals who are embarking on the same wellness journey. It's a space where you can share your personal experiences, triumphs, and challenges, and also learn from others' experiences.

Plus, it's not just a community — it's a vast resource. You'll gain access to insider tips, recipe ideas, motivational stories, and expert advice from experienced like-mind followers. To become part of our thriving Facebook group, simply search 'Diabetes & Low Glycemic Nutrition Information' on Facebook, and hit 'Join'. We can't wait to welcome you to our community and watch you thrive on your Healthy Lifestyle journey!"

GET 4 BONUSES:

Trackers, Planners & Chea Sheets

Diabetes A Comprehensive Quick Guide
Book 1
Best Selling Amazon Author

Exercise For Diabetes
Book 2
Best Selling Amazon Author

AUDIO BOOKS

TRACKERS
WORKBOOKS
AUDIOBOOKS
VIDEO COURSES
TOTAL VALUE: $250 FOR **FREE!**

GET YOUR 4 BONUSES **SCAN ME!**

BONUS 1 OF 4- TRACKERS

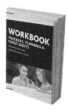

Trackers,
Planners & Cheat
Sheets

This is a set of comprehensive tools designed to help you monitor and track your health metrics. These trackers make it easy to record and understand your diabetes levels, cholesterol counts, and kidney function over time. They are essential aids for anyone seeking to take proactive control of their health and wellness.

Value: $99 - Cost **Free!**

QR Code Below

BONUS 2 OF 4- WORKBOOK

Diabetes A
Comprehensive
Quick Guide
Book 1
Best Selling Amazon Author

Exercise For
Diabetes
Book 2
Best Selling Amazon Author

This essential workbook provides expert advice and practical exercises to manage diabetes, cholesterol, and kidney health, serving as a comprehensive tool for improved wellness.

Value: $51- Cost **Free!**

QR Code Below

BONUS 3 OF 4- AUDIOBOOKS

- CHINESE HERBS
- HOW TO BOOST YOUR METABOLISM
- HOW TO LOSE 10 POUNDS NATURALLY
- NATURAL REMEDIES
- HEALTHY WEIGHTLOSS FOR TEENS

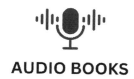

AUDIO BOOKS

Value: $60- Cost **Free!**

QR Code Below

BONUS 4 OF 4- VIDEO COURSE

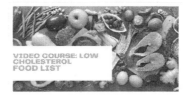

This video course is a comprehensive guide to foods and dietary habits that reduce cholesterol levels, offering tips from experts and serving as your go-to resource for a low-cholesterol lifestyle.

Value: $40- Cost **Free!**

QR Code Below

GET 4 BONUSES:

TRACKERS
WORKBOOKS
AUDIOBOOKS
VIDEO COURSES

TOTAL VALUE: $250 FOR **FREE!**

SCAN THE QR CODE!

MASTERSHIP BOOKS

UK | USA | Canada | Ireland | Australia
India | New Zealand | South Africa | China
Mastership Books is part of the United Arts Publishing
House group of companies based in London, England, UK.
First published by Mastership Books (London, UK), 2023
Text Copyright © United Arts Publishing

Cover design by Rich © United Arts Publishing (UK)
Text and internal design by Rich © United Arts Publishing
(UK)
Image credits reserved.
Color separation by Spitting Image Design Studio
Printed and bound in Great Britain
National Publications Association of Britain
London, England, United Kingdom.
Paper design UAP
A723.5
Title: Low Cholesterol Food List
Design, Bound & Printed:
London, England,
Great Britain.

FREE BOOK CLUB

Email me:
juliameadowsauthor@gmail.com

CONTENTS

INTRODUCTION

Is it safe to say that you are searching for a definitive manual for grasping cholesterol and figuring out which food varieties are useful or hurtful for your well-being? If so, look no further than The Complete Guide to Cholesterol: Low Cholesterol Foods and High Cholesterol Foods to Avoid. Equipped with information from this book, you will want to settle on better decisions to keep your heart sound. With straightforward clarifications and basic ways to integrate the right food varieties into your eating regimen, this book will furnish you with the instruments to oversee and screen your cholesterol levels into the indefinite future. It is the ideal opportunity to assume command over your well-being and get everything rolling to better cholesterol the executives.

Understanding the impact of different foods is essential in maintaining a healthy heart and managing cholesterol levels.

This book, "The Complete Guide to Cholesterol: Low Cholesterol Foods and High Cholesterol Foods to Avoid," is your exhaustive asset for building a heart-solid eating regimen. We will explore an extensive list of low-cholesterol foods across various categories and high-cholesterol foods to limit or avoid. By pursuing informed decisions, you can assume command over your cholesterol levels and advance cardiovascular prosperity.

Lisa is a 45-year-old woman recently diagnosed with high cholesterol levels during a routine medical check-up. She is concerned about her heart health and is motivated to make positive changes to her diet to lower her cholesterol naturally. Lisa is health-conscious and actively seeks information and resources to guide her in making better food choices.

Lisa is frustrated and overwhelmed with the conflicting information about cholesterol and its impact on heart health. She wants a comprehensive resource that clearly understands low- and high-cholesterol foods to avoid and practical guidance on incorporating these changes into her daily meals.

"The Complete Guide to Cholesterol: Low Cholesterol Foods and High Cholesterol Foods to Avoid" is a complete book that is a commonsense asset for people like Lisa who hope to further develop their heart well-being by embracing a low cholesterol diet. The book provides a detailed list of low-cholesterol foods, offers guidance on meal planning, and highlights high-cholesterol foods to avoid.

Its goal is to provide readers with the information and resources they need to make informed food choices and encourage heart-healthy eating habits.

Lisa's journey towards better cholesterol management has been greatly aided by The Complete Guide to Cholesterol: Low Cholesterol Foods and High Cholesterol Foods to Avoid. She knows that with informed choices, she can easily monitor her cholesterol levels and keep her heart healthy for many years. From finding a comprehensive list of low-cholesterol foods to understanding which high-cholesterol foods are best avoided, Lisa has everything he needs for effective healthy lifestyle changes. Indeed, the key to successful management of cholesterol levels is knowledge – and this book provides it in spades!

Lisa's story shows that taking control of one's health starts with making smart decisions about food. You, too, can make informed choices that will keep your heart healthy. So, start reading now and start on your path towards better cholesterol management today!

Shocking Facts...

Did you know cholesterol levels over 200mg/dL are considered high and can jeopardize your coronary illness? According to the American Heart Association, anything above 240 mg/dL is very high.

Then again, assuming your cholesterol levels are excessively low (under 160-180 mg/dl), it could prompt an expanded gamble of stroke and passing because of unfortunate dissemination.

It's vital to note that various sorts of dietary fat affect one's cholesterol levels; immersed fats increment complete cholesterol, while monounsaturated and polyunsaturated fats lower LDL and raise HDL.

The Complete Guide to Cholesterol: Low Cholesterol Foods and High Cholesterol Foods to Avoid is your comprehensive resource for understanding cholesterol and building a heart-healthy diet. With this book, you can confidently pursue more brilliant decisions to guarantee that your cholesterol levels stay in line and your body stays sound.

This book is for you...

The Complete Guide to Cholesterol: Low Cholesterol Foods and High Cholesterol Foods to Avoid is for you whether you're trying to prevent heart disease or want to be sure your overall cholesterol levels are balanced. The many types of cholesterol and how various meals impact them are extensively covered in this book. You'll realize which food varieties are advantageous or hurtful for your well-being and get straightforward clarifications with basic ways to integrate the right food sources into your eating routine.

With this book, you can settle on informed decisions with certainty about what food sources will assist with keeping your heart sound. It's always okay to start making lifestyle changes that promote better cardiovascular well-being - so get started!

With The Complete Guide to Cholesterol, you can take charge of your health and begin taking better care of your cholesterol: Low Cholesterol Food varieties and Elevated Cholesterol Food sources to Keep away from.

Skeptics Read This...

With regard to embracing a solid way of life, if you're skeptical, The Complete Guide to Cholesterol: Low Cholesterol Foods and High Cholesterol Foods to Avoid is the book for you. With straightforward clarifications and basic ways to integrate the right food sources into your eating regimen, this book gives per-users dependable data on cholesterol levels and ways of overseeing them.

This book provides insight into how different types of dietary fat affect cholesterol levels and offers advice about which food varieties should be avoided or limited. By understanding what foods are beneficial or harmful for maintaining heart health, skeptics can become more informed about their cholesterol levels and make better decisions about what they eat.

The Complete Guide to Cholesterol is your comprehensive resource for understanding cholesterol and building a heart-healthy diet. With this book, you can settle on more brilliant decisions with certainty to guarantee that your cholesterol levels stay in line and your body stays solid.

How this book is different...

The Complete Guide to Cholesterol: Low Cholesterol Foods and High Cholesterol Foods to Avoid differs from other diet books because it makes managing cholesterol levels easy. With simple-to-understand guidelines and explanations of how various dietary fats impact cholesterol levels, it has a comprehensive list of Low Cholesterol Foods and High Cholesterol Foods to Avoid justification for why this book gives per-users dependable data that can be utilized to settle on better conclusions about their eating regimens.

This book offers tips for following a heart-healthy diet. It provides insight into understanding food labels and ingredient lists so that readers can easily identify foods beneficial or harmful for managing cholesterol levels. With this knowledge, they can confidently and intelligently select food items from the grocery store or restaurant menus.

How to read this book...

The Complete Guide to Cholesterol: Low Cholesterol Foods and High Cholesterol Foods to Avoid is organized into three sections that provide readers with comprehensive information on managing cholesterol levels. The impact of various dietary fat types on total cholesterol levels is briefly discussed in the first section.

The second section offers practical guidance for adhering to a heart-healthy diet and lists items with low and high cholesterol that should be avoided.

It offers pointers for deciphering ingredient lists, portion measurements, and food labels.

Finally, the third section offers easy-to-follow recipes for delicious meals that are low in cholesterol but still offer plenty of taste and nutrition. These parts will assist perusers with settling on more brilliant decisions about what they eat and fabricating a heart-sound eating routine that can hold their cholesterol levels under tight restraints.

This present time is the ideal opportunity to begin understanding this book because it has become clear how to do so. With The Complete Guide to Cholesterol: Low Cholesterol Foods and High Cholesterol Foods to Avoid, you can start taking better care of your cholesterol levels and continue living a better life. So, stand by no more extended - begin understanding today!

1

UNDERSTANDING CHOLESTEROL AND ITS IMPACT

Explaining cholesterol and its role in the body

Cholesterol is a waxy substance normally tracked down in the body and is significant in making cell layers, delivering chemicals, and helping to process. Your cholesterol is still in the air by two primary sources: cholesterol from food and cholesterol your body makes.

Consuming foods high in saturated or trans-fat raises your LDL (bad) cholesterol levels. This poor cholesterol can contribute to plaque buildup on the artery walls, resulting in heart disease or stroke. However, consuming a diet rich in unsaturated fats can lower LDL levels while raising HDL (good) cholesterol levels.

It is essential to comprehend how various dietary fats affect total cholesterol levels.

It's likewise critical to get ordinary cholesterol screenings at your PCP's office with the goal that you can oversee and follow your levels over the long run.

Other elements, including your age, weight, level of exercise, stress levels, and smoking habits, might all impact the quantity and type of cholesterol in your blood. You may adjust your lifestyle to enhance your overall heart health by knowing how these factors affect your cholesterol levels.

Finding a healthy balance between the two is crucial. By understanding how different dietary fats affect total cholesterol levels and making smart choices when selecting food items, you can take control of your health and well-being. The Complete Guide to Cholesterol: Low Cholesterol Foods and High Cholesterol Foods to Avoid gives you the information you need to make wise choices and create a heart-healthy diet that will help control your cholesterol levels.

Differentiating between LDL (bad) cholesterol and HDL (good) cholesterol

A bad LDL (low-density lipoprotein) can clog arteries and prevent blood from reaching the heart. Foods high in saturated or trans fats increase LDL levels, so limiting these types of fat in your diet is important.

On the other hand, HDL (high-density lipoprotein) cholesterol, is regarded as beneficial because it aids in the removal of excess bad cholesterol from artery walls and transports it back to the liver for elimination. Eating food varieties high in monounsaturated and polyunsaturated fats helps increment HDL levels, making them a significant piece of a heart-solid eating routine.

Knowing what different dietary fats mean for HDL and LDL levels not just assists you with settling on informed conclusions about what to eat and guarantees that your cholesterol levels are overseen and followed over the long haul.

UNDERSTANDING the health risks associated with high cholesterol levels

Your risk for heart disease, stroke, and other serious cardiovascular disorders might rise if your cholesterol levels are high. Various symptoms, including chest discomfort or shortness of breath, can be brought on by the buildup of poor cholesterol on the artery walls, which limits blood flow to the heart. The risk for these complications increases if HDL levels are low and LDL levels are high, so it's important to make lifestyle changes that help keep both in balance.

As well as following a sound eating routine, getting customary activity, stopping smoking, and overseeing feelings of anxiety can all assist with decreasing your gamble of creating complexities because of elevated cholesterol. Working with a specialist to screen cholesterol levels over the long run is likewise significant in recognizing any expected issues and doing whatever it takes to address them.

High cholesterol can be dangerous, but you can make informed decisions about what to eat by understanding how different foods affect your total cholesterol levels.

Additionally, seeing your doctor before beginning any new supplements or drugs that promise to lower cholesterol levels is crucial. While some drugs, like statins, might help lower LDL levels, improper use can have substantial negative effects. It's also crucial to remember that some natural components and herbs may impact your blood sugar and cholesterol levels, so make sure to speak with your doctor before using any of these treatments.

RECOGNIZING the importance of a balanced diet for cholesterol management

A well-balanced diet is essential to control cholesterol levels and lower the gamble of coronary illness and stroke. Food varieties high in unsaturated fats, like olive oil, nuts, seeds, avocados, and greasy fish, are significant for expanding HDL (great) cholesterol while diminishing LDL (terrible) cholesterol. Eating a lot of new products of the soil alongside entire grain food varieties likewise assists hold with adding up to cholesterol levels under wraps.

As well as following a solid eating routine, getting standard active work is significant. Exercise helps increase HDL levels while decreasing LDL levels, so include at least 30 minutes of moderate physical activity daily. Stopping smoking can likewise assist with decreasing the gamble of cardiovascular inconveniences related to elevated cholesterol.

By understanding how cholesterol functions and consolidating a solid eating regimen, actual work, and stress the board into your way of life, you can assume command over your heart's well-being. The Complete Guide to Cholesterol: Low Cholesterol Foods and High Cholesterol Foods to Avoid gives the information needed to assist you in making well-informed eating selections that will lower your cholesterol.

It's also important to remember that alcohol consumption should be limited when managing cholesterol levels. Triglycerides, which are blood fats, and LDL (bad) cholesterol are increased by excessive alcohol consumption. So, stay with moderate drinking propensities if you decide to drink, and consistently check with your PCP before beginning any new dietary changes.

By following a fair eating routine, getting customary actual work, stopping smoking, and restricting liquor consumption, you can develop your cholesterol levels and assume command over your heart's well-being.

By rolling out little improvements, for example, trading out undesirable fats for solid ones or adding more leafy foods into feasts, it's feasible to begin seeing enhancements in your cholesterol levels within only half a month — possibly diminishing your gamble for cardiovascular-related difficulties.

THE LOW CHOLESTEROL FOODS LIST

Fruits and Vegetables:

Apples (1 medium apple):
Cholesterol: 0mg
Sodium: 0mg

BERRIES (1 CUP, mixed berries):
Cholesterol: 0mg
Sodium: 1mg

CITRUS FRUITS (1 MEDIUM ORANGE):
Cholesterol: 0mg
Sodium: 0mg

LEAFY GREENS (1 CUP, raw spinach):
Cholesterol: 0mg
Sodium: 24mg

CRUCIFEROUS VEGETABLES (1 CUP, raw broccoli florets):
   Cholesterol: 0mg
   Sodium: 30mg

TOMATOES (1 MEDIUM TOMATO):
   Cholesterol: 0mg
   Sodium: 6mg

BELL PEPPERS (1 MEDIUM PEPPER):
   Cholesterol: 0mg
   Sodium: 3mg

SWEET POTATOES (1 medium sweet potato):
   Cholesterol: 0mg
   Sodium: 41mg

AVOCADO (1/2 MEDIUM AVOCADO):
   Cholesterol: 0mg
   Sodium: 5mg

PEARS (1 MEDIUM-SIZED FRUIT):
   Cholesterol: 0mg
   Sodium: 0mg

CHERRIES (1 CUP):
   Cholesterol: 0mg
   Sodium: 0mg

. . .

PINEAPPLE (1 CUP, chunks):
Cholesterol: 0mg
Sodium: 2mg

KIWI (1 MEDIUM-SIZED FRUIT):
Cholesterol: 0mg
Sodium: 3mg

PAPAYA (1 CUP, cubes):
Cholesterol: 0mg
Sodium: 8mg

WATERMELON (1 CUP, diced):
Cholesterol: 0mg
Sodium: 2mg

MANGO (1 MEDIUM-SIZED FRUIT):
Cholesterol: 0mg
Sodium: 2mg

PLUMS (1 MEDIUM-SIZED FRUIT):
Cholesterol: 0mg
Sodium: 0mg

GRAPES (1 CUP):

Cholesterol: 0mg
Sodium: 2mg

MELONS (E.G., cantaloupe, honeydew) (1 cup, diced):
Cholesterol: 0mg
Sodium: 18mg

CUCUMBERS (1 CUP, sliced):
Cholesterol: 0mg
Sodium: 2mg

ZUCCHINI (1 CUP, sliced):
Cholesterol: 0mg
Sodium: 6mg

CARROTS (1 MEDIUM-SIZED CARROT):
Cholesterol: 0mg
Sodium: 42mg

EGGPLANT (1 CUP, cubed):
Cholesterol: 0mg
Sodium: 2mg

ASPARAGUS (1 CUP):
Cholesterol: 0mg
Sodium: 2mg

. . .

ARTICHOKES (1 MEDIUM-SIZED ARTICHOKE):
  Cholesterol: 0mg
  Sodium: 76mg

RADISHES (1 CUP, sliced):
  Cholesterol: 0mg
  Sodium: 29mg

SPINACH (1 CUP, raw):
  Cholesterol: 0mg
  Sodium: 24mg

CAULIFLOWER (1 CUP, chopped):
  Cholesterol: 0mg
  Sodium: 30mg

BRUSSELS SPROUTS (1 CUP):
  Cholesterol: 0mg
  Sodium: 15mg

APRICOTS (1 MEDIUM-SIZED FRUIT):
  Cholesterol: 0mg
  Sodium: 1mg

PEACHES (1 MEDIUM-SIZED FRUIT):
  Cholesterol: 0mg
  Sodium: 0mg

. . .

NECTARINES (1 MEDIUM-SIZED FRUIT):
Cholesterol: 0mg
Sodium: 0mg

PLUOTS (1 MEDIUM-SIZED FRUIT):
Cholesterol: 0mg
Sodium: 0mg

GUAVA (1 MEDIUM-SIZED FRUIT):
Cholesterol: 0mg
Sodium: 3mg

PERSIMMONS (1 MEDIUM-SIZED FRUIT):
Cholesterol: 0mg
Sodium: 0mg

CRANBERRIES (1 CUP, whole):
Cholesterol: 0mg
Sodium: 2mg

BLACKBERRIES (1 CUP):
Cholesterol: 0mg
Sodium: 1mg

RASPBERRIES (1 CUP):

Cholesterol: 0mg
Sodium: 0mg

BLUEBERRIES (1 CUP):
Cholesterol: 0mg
Sodium: 1mg

CELERY (1 MEDIUM-SIZED STALK):
Cholesterol: 0mg
Sodium: 32mg

BROCCOLI (1 CUP, chopped):
Cholesterol: 0mg
Sodium: 30mg

BOK CHOY (1 CUP, shredded):
Cholesterol: 0mg
Sodium: 9mg

GREEN BEANS (1 CUP):
Cholesterol: 0mg
Sodium: 6mg

SWISS CHARD (1 CUP, chopped):
Cholesterol: 0mg
Sodium: 77mg

. . .

KALE (1 CUP, chopped):
  Cholesterol: 0mg
  Sodium: 29mg

OKRA (1 CUP, sliced):
  Cholesterol: 0mg
  Sodium: 7mg

CABBAGE (1 CUP, shredded):
  Cholesterol: 0mg
  Sodium: 18mg

COLLARD GREENS (1 CUP, chopped):
  Cholesterol: 0mg
  Sodium: 15mg

TURNIPS (1 MEDIUM-SIZED TURNIP):
  Cholesterol: 0mg
  Sodium: 39mg

FIGS (1 MEDIUM-SIZED FRUIT):
  Cholesterol: 0mg
  Sodium: 0mg

KIWIFRUIT (1 MEDIUM-SIZED FRUIT):
  Cholesterol: 0mg
  Sodium: 2mg

. . .

LYCHEE (1 CUP):
Cholesterol: 0mg
Sodium: 1mg

PASSION FRUIT (1 MEDIUM-SIZED FRUIT):
Cholesterol: 0mg
Sodium: 0mg

STARFRUIT (1 MEDIUM-SIZED FRUIT):
Cholesterol: 0mg
Sodium: 2mg

MULBERRIES (1 CUP):
Cholesterol: 0mg
Sodium: 10mg

GOJI BERRIES (1 OZ):
Cholesterol: 0mg
Sodium: 75mg

POMEGRANATE (1 MEDIUM-SIZED FRUIT):
Cholesterol: 0mg
Sodium: 3mg

CHERIMOYA (1 MEDIUM-SIZED FRUIT):

Cholesterol: 0mg
Sodium: 7mg

QUINCE (1 MEDIUM-SIZED FRUIT):
Cholesterol: 0mg
Sodium: 1mg

SNOW PEAS (1 CUP):
Cholesterol: 0mg
Sodium: 4mg

JICAMA (1 CUP, sliced):
Cholesterol: 0mg
Sodium: 4mg

LEEKS (1 CUP, sliced):
Cholesterol: 0mg
Sodium: 36mg

WATERCRESS (1 CUP):
Cholesterol: 0mg
Sodium: 79mg

BAMBOO SHOOTS (1 CUP, sliced):
Cholesterol: 0mg
Sodium: 1mg

· · ·

DAIKON RADISH (1 CUP, sliced):
    Cholesterol: 0mg
    Sodium: 27mg

KOHLRABI (1 CUP, cubes):
    Cholesterol: 0mg
    Sodium: 36mg

ENDIVE (1 CUP, chopped):
    Cholesterol: 0mg
    Sodium: 22mg

RUTABAGA (1 CUP, cubes):
    Cholesterol: 0mg
    Sodium: 52mg

MUSTARD GREENS (1 CUP, chopped):
    Cholesterol: 0mg
    Sodium: 13mg

ELDERBERRIES (1 CUP):
    Cholesterol: 0mg
    Sodium: 1mg

GOOSEBERRIES (1 CUP):
    Cholesterol: 0mg
    Sodium: 2mg

. . .

BOYSENBERRIES (I CUP):
    Cholesterol: 0mg
    Sodium: 1mg

CURRANTS (BLACK, red, or white) (I cup):
    Cholesterol: 0mg
    Sodium: 2mg

TANGERINES (I MEDIUM-SIZED FRUIT):
    Cholesterol: 0mg
    Sodium: 1mg

MULBERRIES (I CUP):
    Cholesterol: 0mg
    Sodium: 3mg

POMELO (I CUP, sections):
    Cholesterol: 0mg
    Sodium: 0mg

CARAMBOLA (STARFRUIT) (I MEDIUM-SIZED FRUIT):
    Cholesterol: 0mg
    Sodium: 2mg

PERSIMMON (I MEDIUM-SIZED FRUIT):

Cholesterol: 0mg
Sodium: 1mg

PLANTAINS (1 MEDIUM-SIZED FRUIT):
Cholesterol: 0mg
Sodium: 2mg

CHAYOTE (1 CUP, sliced):
Cholesterol: 0mg
Sodium: 2mg

CELERIAC (CELERY ROOT) (1 CUP, sliced):
Cholesterol: 0mg
Sodium: 98mg

HUBBARD SQUASH (1 CUP, mashed):
Cholesterol: 0mg
Sodium: 8mg

ESCAROLE (1 CUP, chopped):
Cholesterol: 0mg
Sodium: 17mg

DANDELION GREENS (1 CUP, chopped):
Cholesterol: 0mg
Sodium: 76mg

• • •

MACHE (LAMB'S LETTUCE) (I CUP):
Cholesterol: 0mg
Sodium: 15mg

FIDDLEHEADS (I CUP):
Cholesterol: 0mg
Sodium: 1mg

WAX BEANS (Yellow beans) (I cup):
Cholesterol: 0mg
Sodium: 1mg

CHARD (SWISS CHARD) (I CUP, chopped):
Cholesterol: 0mg
Sodium: 77mg

ZUCCHINI BLOSSOMS (3 BLOSSOMS):
Cholesterol: 0mg
Sodium: 0mg

LOGANBERRIES (I CUP):
Cholesterol: 0mg
Sodium: 0mg

MARIONBERRIES (I CUP):
Cholesterol: 0mg
Sodium: 0mg

. . .

BOYSENBERRIES (1 CUP):
Cholesterol: 0mg
Sodium: 0mg

HUCKLEBERRIES (1 CUP):
Cholesterol: 0mg
Sodium: 2mg

QUINCE (1 MEDIUM-SIZED FRUIT):
Cholesterol: 0mg
Sodium: 1mg

CRABAPPLE (1 MEDIUM-SIZED FRUIT):
Cholesterol: 0mg
Sodium: 1mg

SASKATOON BERRIES (1 CUP):
Cholesterol: 0mg
Sodium: 0mg

UGLI FRUIT (1 MEDIUM-SIZED FRUIT):
Cholesterol: 0mg
Sodium: 0mg

FEIJOA (1 MEDIUM-SIZED FRUIT):

Cholesterol: 0mg
Sodium: 0mg

PAWPAW (1 MEDIUM-SIZED FRUIT):
Cholesterol: 0mg
Sodium: 0mg

WATER CHESTNUTS (1 CUP, sliced):
Cholesterol: 0mg
Sodium: 11mg

FENNEL (1 CUP, sliced):
Cholesterol: 0mg
Sodium: 45mg

ROMANESCO (1 CUP, chopped):
Cholesterol: 0mg
Sodium: 30mg

CHIVES (1 TABLESPOON, chopped):
Cholesterol: 0mg
Sodium: 0mg

SORREL (1 CUP, chopped):
Cholesterol: 0mg
Sodium: 10mg

. . .

TATSOI (1 CUP, **chopped**):
    Cholesterol: 0mg
    Sodium: 13mg

MIZUNA (1 CUP, **chopped**):
    Cholesterol: 0mg
    Sodium: 15mg

ARROWHEAD (CHINESE WATER **spinach**) (1 **cup, chopped**):
    Cholesterol: 0mg
    Sodium: 34mg

GARLIC SCAPES (1 CUP, **chopped**):
    Cholesterol: 0mg
    Sodium: 1mg

WATER CHESTNUTS (1 CUP, **sliced**):
    Cholesterol: 0mg
    Sodium: 4mg

HORNED **melon (Kiwano)** (1 **medium-sized fruit**):
    Cholesterol: 0mg
    Sodium: 2mg

TAMARILLO (TREE TOMATO) (1 **medium-sized fruit**):
    Cholesterol: 0mg
    Sodium: 2mg

. . .

RAMBUTAN (1 CUP):
    Cholesterol: 0mg
    Sodium: 2mg

ACEROLA (BARBADOS CHERRY) (1 CUP):
    Cholesterol: 0mg
    Sodium: 7mg

BREADFRUIT (1 CUP, sliced):
    Cholesterol: 0mg
    Sodium: 2mg

JACKFRUIT (1 CUP, sliced):
    Cholesterol: 0mg
    Sodium: 3mg

LYCHEE (1 CUP):
    Cholesterol: 0mg
    Sodium: 1mg

UGNI (CHILEAN GUAVA) (1 CUP):
    Cholesterol: 0mg
    Sodium: 0mg

LONGAN (1 CUP):

Cholesterol: 0mg
Sodium: 1mg

MIRACLE FRUIT (1 BERRY):
Cholesterol: 0mg
Sodium: 0mg

CHINESE BROCCOLI (GAI LAN) (1 cup, chopped):
Cholesterol: 0mg
Sodium: 60mg

RAPINI (BROCCOLI RABE) (1 CUP, chopped):
Cholesterol: 0mg
Sodium: 210mg

MIZUNA (1 CUP, chopped):
Cholesterol: 0mg
Sodium: 13mg

AMARANTH LEAVES (1 CUP, cooked):
Cholesterol: 0mg
Sodium: 4mg

WATER SPINACH (KANGKONG) (1 CUP, cooked):
Cholesterol: 0mg
Sodium: 17mg

. . .

WINGED BEANS (GOA beans) (1 cup, sliced):
Cholesterol: 0mg
Sodium: 1mg

DULSE (RED SEAWEED) (1 OZ):
Cholesterol: 0mg
Sodium: 69mg

Whole Grains:

Oats (1 cup cooked):
Cholesterol: 0mg
Sodium: 2mg

QUINOA (1 CUP COOKED):
Cholesterol: 0mg
Sodium: 13mg

BROWN RICE (1 CUP COOKED):
Cholesterol: 0mg
Sodium: 1mg

BARLEY (1 CUP COOKED):
Cholesterol: 0mg
Sodium: 4mg

WHOLE WHEAT BREAD (1 SLICE):
Cholesterol: 0mg

Sodium: 130mg

WHOLE WHEAT PASTA (1 cup cooked):
Cholesterol: 0mg
Sodium: 1mg

BUCKWHEAT (1 CUP COOKED):
Cholesterol: 0mg
Sodium: 1mg

MILLET (1 CUP COOKED):
Cholesterol: 0mg
Sodium: 2mg

FARRO (1 CUP COOKED):
Cholesterol: 0mg
Sodium: 0mg

BULGUR (1 CUP COOKED):
Cholesterol: 0mg
Sodium: 6mg

AMARANTH (1 CUP COOKED):
Cholesterol: 0mg
Sodium: 4mg

. . .

TEFF (I CUP COOKED):
Cholesterol: 0mg
Sodium: 4mg

SORGHUM (I CUP COOKED):
Cholesterol: 0mg
Sodium: 3mg

FREEKEH (I CUP COOKED):
Cholesterol: 0mg
Sodium: 8mg

SPELT (I CUP COOKED):
Cholesterol: 0mg
Sodium: 6mg

KAMUT (I CUP COOKED):
Cholesterol: 0mg
Sodium: 2mg

WILD RICE (I CUP COOKED):
Cholesterol: 0mg
Sodium: 7mg

RYE (I CUP COOKED):
Cholesterol: 0mg
Sodium: 2mg

. . .

QUINOA FLAKES (I CUP COOKED):
    Cholesterol: 0mg
    Sodium: 1mg

FONIO (I CUP COOKED):
    Cholesterol: 0mg
    Sodium: 5mg

JOB'S TEARS (Coix) (I cup cooked):
    Cholesterol: 0mg
    Sodium: 2mg

EINKORN (I CUP COOKED):
    Cholesterol: 0mg
    Sodium: 2mg

EMMER (I CUP COOKED):
    Cholesterol: 0mg
    Sodium: 0mg

TRITICALE (I CUP COOKED):
    Cholesterol: 0mg
    Sodium: 2mg

BLACK RICE (FORBIDDEN Rice) (I cup cooked):

Cholesterol: 0mg
Sodium: 4mg

RED RICE (1 CUP COOKED):
Cholesterol: 0mg
Sodium: 10mg

SPELT FLAKES (1 CUP COOKED):
Cholesterol: 0mg
Sodium: 0mg

KANIWA (1 CUP COOKED):
Cholesterol: 0mg
Sodium: 1mg

Lean proteins:

Skinless Chicken

Chicken Breast (boneless, skinless - 3 oz serving):
Cholesterol: 85mg
Sodium: 74mg

CHICKEN TENDERLOINS (SKINLESS - 3 oz serving):
Cholesterol: 85mg
Sodium: 74mg

. . .

CHICKEN THIGH (BONELESS, skinless - 3 oz serving):
Cholesterol: 82mg
Sodium: 74mg

CHICKEN DRUMSTICK (BONELESS, skinless - 3 oz serving):
Cholesterol: 80mg
Sodium: 71mg

CHICKEN WING (BONELESS, skinless - 3 oz serving):
Cholesterol: 77mg
Sodium: 74mg

CHICKEN FILLET (SKINLESS - 3 oz serving):
Cholesterol: 85mg
Sodium: 74mg

CHICKEN CUTLET (SKINLESS - 3 oz serving):
Cholesterol: 85mg
Sodium: 74mg

CHICKEN STRIP (SKINLESS - 3 oz serving):
Cholesterol: 85mg
Sodium: 74mg

CHICKEN TENDERS (SKINLESS - 3 oz serving):
Cholesterol: 85mg
Sodium: 74mg

. . .

CHICKEN SLICES (SKINLESS - 3 oz serving):
Cholesterol: 85mg
Sodium: 74mg

CHICKEN MEDALLIONS (SKINLESS - 3 oz serving):
Cholesterol: 85mg
Sodium: 74mg

Turkey Breast

Boneless, Skinless Turkey Breast (3 oz serving):
Cholesterol: 26mg
Sodium: 45mg

TURKEY BREAST TENDERLOINS (3 oz serving):
Cholesterol: 27mg
Sodium: 40mg

TURKEY BREAST CUTLETS (3 oz serving):
Cholesterol: 26mg
Sodium: 46mg

TURKEY BREAST FILLETS (3 oz serving):
Cholesterol: 27mg
Sodium: 44mg

. . .

TURKEY BREAST SLICES (3 oz serving):
Cholesterol: 27mg
Sodium: 47mg

TURKEY BREAST ROAST (without skin - 3 oz serving):
Cholesterol: 26mg
Sodium: 55mg

GROUND TURKEY BREAST (LEAN, without skin - 3 oz serving):
Cholesterol: 57mg
Sodium: 71mg

Fish

Cod (3 oz serving):
Cholesterol: 45mg
Sodium: 63mg

HADDOCK (3 OZ SERVING):
Cholesterol: 60mg
Sodium: 74mg

FLOUNDER (3 OZ SERVING):
Cholesterol: 49mg
Sodium: 90mg

SOLE (3 OZ SERVING):

Cholesterol: 63mg
Sodium: 70mg

TILAPIA (3 OZ SERVING):
Cholesterol: 37mg
Sodium: 44mg

RAINBOW TROUT (3 OZ SERVING):
Cholesterol: 61mg
Sodium: 49mg

STEELHEAD TROUT (3 OZ SERVING):
Cholesterol: 59mg
Sodium: 47mg

ATLANTIC MACKEREL (3 OZ SERVING):
Cholesterol: 18mg
Sodium: 93mg

PACIFIC MACKEREL (3 OZ SERVING):
Cholesterol: 17mg
Sodium: 88mg

WHITEFISH (3 OZ SERVING):
Cholesterol: 60mg
Sodium: 51mg

.　.　.

LAKE TROUT (3 OZ SERVING):
    Cholesterol: 62mg
    Sodium: 55mg

ARCTIC CHAR (3 OZ SERVING):
    Cholesterol: 46mg
    Sodium: 54mg

MAHI-MAHI (DORADO) (3 OZ SERVING):
    Cholesterol: 57mg
    Sodium: 135mg

GROUPER (3 OZ SERVING):
    Cholesterol: 59mg
    Sodium: 75mg

RED SNAPPER (3 OZ SERVING):
    Cholesterol: 64mg
    Sodium: 63mg

YELLOWTAIL SNAPPER (3 OZ SERVING):
    Cholesterol: 57mg
    Sodium: 71m

COBIA (3 OZ SERVING):
    Cholesterol: 37mg
    Sodium: 78mg

. . .

PANGASIUS (SWAI) (3 OZ SERVING):
    Cholesterol: 49mg
    Sodium: 54mg

ALASKAN SALMON (3 OZ SERVING):
    Cholesterol: 54mg
    Sodium: 45mg

CHINOOK SALMON (3 OZ SERVING):
    Cholesterol: 47mg
    Sodium: 47mg

SOCKEYE SALMON (3 OZ SERVING):
    Cholesterol: 59mg
    Sodium: 60mg

CHUM SALMON (3 OZ SERVING):
    Cholesterol: 57mg
    Sodium: 48mg

Shellfish

Crab (3 oz serving):
    Cholesterol: 42mg
    Sodium: 324mg

. . .

CLAMS **(3 OZ SERVING):**
    Cholesterol: 48mg
    Sodium: 126mg

MUSSELS **(3 OZ SERVING):**
    Cholesterol: 48mg
    Sodium: 367mg

SCALLOPS **(3 OZ SERVING):**
    Cholesterol: 35mg
    Sodium: 267mg

OYSTERS **(3 OZ SERVING):**
    Cholesterol: 49mg
    Sodium: 195mg

CRAWFISH **(**CRAYFISH**) (3 OZ SERVING):**
    Cholesterol: 50mg
    Sodium: 189mg

OCTOPUS **(3 OZ SERVING):**
    Cholesterol: 48mg
    Sodium: 351mg

COCKLES **(3 OZ SERVING):**
    Cholesterol: 50mg
    Sodium: 148mg

. . .

CONCH (3 OZ SERVING):
    Cholesterol: 40mg
    Sodium: 144mg

PERIWINKLES (3 OZ SERVING):
    Cholesterol: 50mg
    Sodium: 220mg

WHELKS (3 OZ SERVING):
    Cholesterol: 50mg
    Sodium: 360mg

RAZOR CLAMS (3 OZ SERVING):
    Cholesterol: 56mg
    Sodium: 148mg

LIMPETS (3 OZ SERVING):
    Cholesterol: 45mg
    Sodium: 88mg

STONE CRAB (3 OZ SERVING):
    Cholesterol: 37mg
    Sodium: 388mg

BAY SCALLOPS (3 OZ SERVING):

Cholesterol: 35mg
Sodium: 541mg

SLIPPER LOBSTER (3 OZ SERVING):
Cholesterol: 56mg
Sodium: 158mg

GREEN CRABS (3 OZ SERVING):
Cholesterol: 54mg
Sodium: 380mg

MANILA CLAMS (3 OZ SERVING):
Cholesterol: 48mg
Sodium: 453mg

SOFTSHELL CLAMS (3 OZ SERVING):
Cholesterol: 25mg
Sodium: 567mg

Legumes

Lentils (1 cup cooked):
Cholesterol: 0mg
Sodium: 2mg

CHICKPEAS (GARBANZO BEANS – 1 cup cooked):
Cholesterol: 0mg
Sodium: 9mg

. . .

BLACK BEANS (I CUP COOKED):
 Cholesterol: 0mg
 Sodium: 1mg

KIDNEY BEANS (I CUP COOKED):
 Cholesterol: 0mg
 Sodium: 1mg

NAVY BEANS (I CUP COOKED):
 Cholesterol: 0mg
 Sodium: 1mg

PINTO BEANS (I CUP COOKED):
 Cholesterol: 0mg
 Sodium: 1mg

CANNELLINI BEANS (I CUP COOKED):
 Cholesterol: 0mg
 Sodium: 4mg

GREAT NORTHERN BEANS (I cup cooked):
 Cholesterol: 0mg
 Sodium: 1mg

LIMA BEANS (I CUP COOKED):

Cholesterol: 0mg
Sodium: 2mg

FAVA BEANS (1 CUP COOKED):
Cholesterol: 0mg
Sodium: 2mg

ADZUKI BEANS (1 CUP COOKED):
Cholesterol: 0mg
Sodium: 1mg

BLACK-EYED PEAS (1 CUP COOKED):
Cholesterol: 0mg
Sodium: 1mg

SPLIT PEAS (1 CUP COOKED):
Cholesterol: 0mg
Sodium: 4mg

GREEN PEAS (1 CUP COOKED):
Cholesterol: 0mg
Sodium: 3mg

MUNG BEANS (1 CUP COOKED):
Cholesterol: 0mg
Sodium: 2mg

. . .

RED LENTILS (1 CUP COOKED):
Cholesterol: 0mg
Sodium: 1mg

GREEN LENTILS (1 CUP COOKED):
Cholesterol: 0mg
Sodium: 1mg

YELLOW LENTILS (1 CUP COOKED):
Cholesterol: 0mg
Sodium: 1mg

FRENCH LENTILS (1 CUP COOKED):
Cholesterol: 0mg
Sodium: 1mg

CRANBERRY BEANS (1 CUP COOKED):
Cholesterol: 0mg
Sodium: 3mg

SOYBEANS (EDAMAME – 1 cup cooked):
Cholesterol: 0mg
Sodium: 8mg

BLACK SOYBEANS (1 CUP COOKED):
Cholesterol: 0mg
Sodium: 1mg

. . .

BUTTER BEANS (LIMA BEANS – 1 cup cooked):
Cholesterol: 0mg
Sodium: 0mg

PEANUTS (1 OZ SERVING):
Cholesterol: 0mg
Sodium: 1mg

COWPEAS (BLACK-EYED COWPEAS – 1 cup cooked):
Cholesterol: 0mg
Sodium: 1mg

CHICKPEA FLOUR (BESAN – 1 cup):
Cholesterol: 0mg
Sodium: 20mg

MOONG DAL (SPLIT MUNG BEANS – 1 cup cooked):
Cholesterol: 0mg
Sodium: 2mg

URAD DAL (BLACK GRAM DAL – 1 cup cooked):
Cholesterol: 0mg
Sodium: 1mg

MASOOR DAL (RED LENTIL DAL – 1 cup cooked):

Cholesterol: 0mg
Sodium: 2mg

RAJMA (RED KIDNEY BEANS – 1 cup cooked):
Cholesterol: 0mg
Sodium: 2mg

CHANA DAL (SPLIT CHICKPEAS – 1 cup cooked):
Cholesterol: 0mg
Sodium: 3mg

YELLOW SPLIT PEAS (1 cup cooked):
Cholesterol: 0mg
Sodium: 0mg

NAVY PEA BEANS (1 cup cooked):
Cholesterol: 0mg
Sodium: 0mg

MUNG BEAN SPROUTS (1 CUP):
Cholesterol: 0mg
Sodium: 6mg

LENTIL SPROUTS (1 CUP):
Cholesterol: 0mg
Sodium: 2mg

. . .

CHICKPEA SPROUTS (1 CUP):
   Cholesterol: 0mg
   Sodium: 8mg

BLACK BEAN SPROUTS (1 CUP):
   Cholesterol: 0mg
   Sodium: 7mg

PEA SPROUTS (1 CUP):
   Cholesterol: 0mg
   Sodium: 2mg

PEA PROTEIN ISOLATE (POWDERED FORM – 1 OZ):
   Cholesterol: 0mg
   Sodium: 251mg

RED BEAN PASTE (SWEETENED – 1 OZ):
   Cholesterol: 0mg
   Sodium: 3mg

WHITE BEAN PASTE (SWEETENED – 1 OZ):
   Cholesterol: 0mg
   Sodium: 6mg

LUPINI BEANS (1 CUP):
   Cholesterol: 0mg
   Sodium: 1mg

. . .

WINGED BEANS (GOA BEANS – 1 cup):
Cholesterol: 0mg
Sodium: 3mg

HYACINTH BEANS (LABLAB BEANS – 1 cup):
Cholesterol: 0mg
Sodium: 2mg

BAMBARA BEANS (VIGNA UBTERRANEAN – 1 cup):
Cholesterol: 0mg
Sodium: 5mg

LENTIL PASTA (MADE from lentil flour – 2 oz):
Cholesterol: 0mg
Sodium: 0mg

CHICKPEA PASTA (MADE from chickpea flour – 2 oz):
Cholesterol: 0mg
Sodium: 0mg

BLACK BEAN PASTA (made of black bean flour – 2 oz):
Cholesterol: 0mg
Sodium: 5mg

SPLIT PEA SOUP (1 CUP):

Cholesterol: omg
Sodium: 653mg

Healthy fats:

Oils

Canola oil (1 tbsp):
Cholesterol: omg
Sodium: omg

OLIVE OIL (1 TBSP):
Cholesterol: omg
Sodium: omg

AVOCADO OIL (1 TBSP):
Cholesterol: omg
Sodium: omg

FLAXSEED OIL (1 TBSP):
Cholesterol: omg
Sodium: omg

PEANUT OIL (1 TBSP):
Cholesterol: omg
Sodium: omg

. . .

SESAME OIL (1 TBSP):
    Cholesterol: 0mg
    Sodium: 0mg

SUNFLOWER OIL (1 TBSP):
    Cholesterol: 0mg
    Sodium: 0mg

SAFFLOWER OIL (1 TBSP):
    Cholesterol: 0mg
    Sodium: 0mg

CORN OIL (1 TBSP):
    Cholesterol: 0mg
    Sodium: 0mg

SOYBEAN OIL (1 TBSP):
    Cholesterol: 0mg
    Sodium: 0mg

RICE BRAN OIL (1 TBSP):
    Cholesterol: 0mg
    Sodium: 0mg

GRAPESEED OIL (1 TBSP):
    Cholesterol: 0mg
    Sodium: 0mg

. . .

WALNUT OIL (I TBSP):
Cholesterol: omg
Sodium: omg

ALMOND OIL (I TBSP):
Cholesterol: omg
Sodium: omg

PISTACHIO OIL (I TBSP):
Cholesterol: omg
Sodium: omg

HAZELNUT OIL (I TBSP):
Cholesterol: omg
Sodium: omg

MACADAMIA NUT OIL (I TBSP):
Cholesterol: omg
Sodium: omg

HEMPSEED OIL (I TBSP):
Cholesterol: omg
Sodium: omg

PUMPKIN SEED OIL (I TBSP):

Cholesterol: omg
Sodium: omg

CAMELINA OIL (1 TBSP):
Cholesterol: omg
Sodium: omg

MUSTARD OIL (1 TBSP):
Cholesterol: omg
Sodium: omg

POPPYSEED OIL (1 TBSP):
Cholesterol: omg
Sodium: omg

PECAN OIL (1 TBSP):
Cholesterol: omg
Sodium: omg

APRICOT KERNEL OIL (1 TBSP):
Cholesterol: omg
Sodium: omg

BORAGE OIL (1 TBSP):
Cholesterol: omg
Sodium: omg

·   ·   ·

BLACK CURRANT SEED oil (1 tbsp):
  Cholesterol: 0mg
  Sodium: 0mg

CHIA SEED OIL (1 TBSP):
  Cholesterol: 0mg
  Sodium: 0mg

EVENING PRIMROSE OIL (1 TBSP):
  Cholesterol: 0mg
  Sodium: 0mg

GOOSEBERRY SEED OIL (1 TBSP):
  Cholesterol: 0mg
  Sodium: 0mg

CRANBERRY SEED OIL (1 TBSP):
  Cholesterol: 0mg
  Sodium: 0mg

KIWI SEED OIL (1 TBSP):
  Cholesterol: 0mg
  Sodium: 0mg

ROSEHIP SEED OIL (1 TBSP):
  Cholesterol: 0mg
  Sodium: 0mg

. . .

SACHA INCHI OIL (I TBSP):
　　Cholesterol: 0mg
　　Sodium: 0mg

SEABUCKTHORN OIL (I TBSP):
　　Cholesterol: 0mg
　　Sodium: 0mg

WATERMELON SEED OIL (I TBSP):
　　Cholesterol: 0mg
　　Sodium: 0mg

TAMANU OIL (I TBSP):
　　Cholesterol: 0mg
　　Sodium: 0mg

BLACK SESAME OIL (I TBSP):
　　Cholesterol: 0mg
　　Sodium: 0mg

MORINGA OIL (I TBSP):
　　Cholesterol: 0mg
　　Sodium: 0mg

POMEGRANATE SEED OIL (I TBSP):

Cholesterol: 0mg
Sodium: 0mg

RASPBERRY SEED OIL (1 TBSP):
    Cholesterol: 0mg
    Sodium: 0mg

BABBASU OIL (1 TBSP):
    Cholesterol: 0mg
    Sodium: 0mg

KARANJA OIL (1 TBSP):
    Cholesterol: 0mg
    Sodium: 0mg

KUKUI NUT OIL (1 TBSP):
    Cholesterol: 0mg
    Sodium: 0mg

MARACUJA OIL (1 TBSP):
    Cholesterol: 0mg
    Sodium: 0mg

NEEM OIL (1 TBSP):
    Cholesterol: 0mg
    Sodium: 0mg

.   .   .

Nigella sativa (Black seed) oil (1 tbsp):
Cholesterol: 0mg
Sodium: 0mg

Papaya seed oil (1 tbsp):
Cholesterol: 0mg
Sodium: 0mg

Tamanu oil (1 tbsp):
Cholesterol: 0mg
Sodium: 0mg

Nuts

Almonds (1 oz serving):
Cholesterol: 0mg
Sodium: 0mg

Cashews (1 oz serving):
Cholesterol: 0mg
Sodium: 3mg

Pistachios (1 oz serving):
Cholesterol: 0mg
Sodium: 0mg

Walnuts (1 oz serving):
Cholesterol: 0mg

Sodium: 0mg

PECANS (1 OZ SERVING):
Cholesterol: 0mg
Sodium: 0mg

HAZELNUTS (1 OZ SERVING):
Cholesterol: 0mg
Sodium: 0mg

MACADAMIA NUTS (1 OZ SERVING):
Cholesterol: 0mg
Sodium: 0mg

BRAZIL NUTS (1 OZ SERVING):
Cholesterol: 0mg
Sodium: 0mg

PINE NUTS (1 OZ SERVING):
Cholesterol: 0mg
Sodium: 0mg

CHESTNUTS (1 OZ SERVING):
Cholesterol: 0mg
Sodium: 0mg

. . .

Peanuts (1 oz serving):
   Cholesterol: 0mg
   Sodium: 1mg

Seeds

Pumpkin seeds (pepitas) (1 oz serving):
   Cholesterol: 0mg
   Sodium: 5mg

Sunflower seeds (1 oz serving):
   Cholesterol: 0mg
   Sodium: 1mg

Hemp seeds (1 oz serving):
   Cholesterol: 0mg
   Sodium: 0mg

Poppy seeds (1 oz serving):
   Cholesterol: 0mg
   Sodium: 2mg

Watermelon seeds (1 oz serving):
   Cholesterol: 0mg
   Sodium: 0mg

Melon seeds (1 oz serving):
   Cholesterol: 0mg

Sodium: 1mg

KIWIFRUIT SEEDS (1 OZ SERVING):
Cholesterol: 0mg
Sodium: 2mg

BLACK SESAME SEEDS (1 OZ serving):
Cholesterol: 0mg
Sodium: 2mg

WHITE SESAME SEEDS (1 OZ serving):
Cholesterol: 0mg
Sodium: 3mg

LINSEEDS (FLAXSEEDS) (1 OZ SERVING):
Cholesterol: 0mg
Sodium: 1mg

POPPY SEEDS (1 OZ SERVING):
Cholesterol: 0mg
Sodium: 2mg

NIGER SEEDS (1 OZ SERVING):
Cholesterol: 0mg
Sodium: 3mg

· · ·

Lotus seeds (phool makhana) (1 oz serving):
Cholesterol: 0mg
Sodium: 0mg

Pili nuts (1 oz serving):
Cholesterol: 0mg
Sodium: 0mg

Tamarind seeds (1 oz serving):
Cholesterol: 0mg
Sodium: 0mg

Lotus nuts (liánzǐ) (1 oz serving):
Cholesterol: 0mg
Sodium: 0mg

Beechnuts (1 oz serving):
Cholesterol: 0mg
Sodium: 0mg

Acorns (1 oz serving):
Cholesterol: 0mg
Sodium: 0mg

Candle nuts (kukui nuts) (1 oz serving):
Cholesterol: 0mg
Sodium: 1mg

. . .

CEMPEDAK SEEDS (I OZ SERVING):
  Cholesterol: omg
  Sodium: omg

WINGED BEAN SEEDS (I oz serving):
  Cholesterol: omg
  Sodium: omg

WALNUT SEEDS (green outer layer) (I oz serving):
  Cholesterol: omg
  Sodium: omg

SHEA NUTS (I OZ SERVING):
  Cholesterol: omg
  Sodium: omg

BERTHOLLETIA EXCELSA (BRAZIL nut seeds) (I oz serving):
  Cholesterol: omg
  Sodium: omg

ALEURITES MOLUCCANA (CANDLENUT seeds) (I oz serving):
  Cholesterol: omg
  Sodium: omg

SAPINDUS MUKOROSSI (SOAPNUT seeds) (I oz serving):

Cholesterol: 0mg
Sodium: 0mg

HMONG CUCUMBER SEEDS (1 oz serving):
Cholesterol: 0mg
Sodium: 0mg

AMAZONIAN COCONUT SEEDS (1 oz serving):
Cholesterol: 0mg
Sodium: 0mg

JUNGLE PEANUTS (1 OZ SERVING):
Cholesterol: 0mg
Sodium: 0mg

SACHA INCHI SEEDS (1 oz serving):
Cholesterol: 0mg
Sodium: 0mg

BLACKBERRY SEEDS (1 OZ SERVING):
Cholesterol: 0mg
Sodium: 0mg

BLUEBERRY SEEDS (1 OZ SERVING):
Cholesterol: 0mg
Sodium: 0mg

. . .

KIWI SEEDS (1 OZ SERVING):
    Cholesterol: omg
    Sodium: omg

PASSION FRUIT SEEDS (1 oz serving):
    Cholesterol: omg
    Sodium: omg

STRAWBERRY SEEDS (1 OZ SERVING):
    Cholesterol: omg
    Sodium: omg

BLACK CURRANT SEEDS (1 oz serving):
    Cholesterol: omg
    Sodium: omg

RASPBERRY SEEDS (1 OZ SERVING):
    Cholesterol: omg
    Sodium: omg

CRANBERRY SEEDS (1 OZ SERVING):
    Cholesterol: omg
    Sodium: omg

GOJI BERRY SEEDS (1 oz serving):
    Cholesterol: omg
    Sodium: omg

. . .

TOMATO SEEDS (1 OZ SERVING):
Cholesterol: 0mg
Sodium: 1mg

GUAVA SEEDS (1 OZ SERVING):
Cholesterol: 0mg
Sodium: 0mg

FIG SEEDS (1 OZ SERVING):
Cholesterol: 0mg
Sodium: 0mg

PEAR SEEDS (1 OZ SERVING):
Cholesterol: 0mg
Sodium: 0mg

PINEAPPLE SEEDS (1 OZ SERVING):
Cholesterol: 0mg
Sodium: 0mg

DRAGON FRUIT SEEDS (1 oz serving):
Cholesterol: 0mg
Sodium: 1mg

AVOCADO SEEDS (EDIBLE; if prepared) (1 oz serving):

Cholesterol: 0mg
Sodium: 0mg

FENNEL SEEDS (1 OZ SERVING):
Cholesterol: 0mg
Sodium: 1mg

FENUGREEK SEEDS (1 OZ SERVING):
Cholesterol: 0mg
Sodium: 7mg

CORIANDER SEEDS (1 OZ SERVING):
Cholesterol: 0mg
Sodium: 3mg

CUMIN SEEDS (1 OZ SERVING):
Cholesterol: 0mg
Sodium: 10mg

MUSTARD SEEDS (1 OZ SERVING):
Cholesterol: 0mg
Sodium: 5mg

CARDAMOM SEEDS (1 OZ SERVING):
Cholesterol: 0mg
Sodium: 0mg

. . .

ANISE SEEDS (I OZ SERVING):
  Cholesterol: 0mg
  Sodium: 1mg

CARAWAY SEEDS (I OZ SERVING):
  Cholesterol: 0mg
  Sodium: 3mg

CELERY SEEDS (I OZ SERVING):
  Cholesterol: 0mg
  Sodium: 95mg

DILL SEEDS (I OZ SERVING):
  Cholesterol: 0mg
  Sodium: 6mg

SACHA INCHI SEEDS (I oz serving):
  Cholesterol: 0mg
  Sodium: 0mg

POMEGRANATE SEEDS (I OZ SERVING):
  Cholesterol: 0mg
  Sodium: 0mg

CUCUMBER SEEDS (I OZ SERVING):
  Cholesterol: 0mg
  Sodium: 1mg

. . .

GRAPE SEEDS (1 OZ SERVING):
Cholesterol: 0mg
Sodium: 1mg

PAPAYA SEEDS (1 OZ SERVING):
Cholesterol: 0mg
Sodium: 0mg

Nut Butter

Almond and cashew butter blend (1 tbsp):
Cholesterol: 0mg
Sodium: 0mg

ALMOND AND WALNUT butter blend (1 tbsp):
Cholesterol: 0mg
Sodium: 0mg

CASHEW & macadamia nut butter blend (1 tbsp):
Cholesterol: 0mg
Sodium: 0mg

PISTACHIO and almond butter blend (1 tbsp):
Cholesterol: 0mg
Sodium: 0mg

. . .

SUNFLOWER AND FLAXSEED **butter blend (1 tbsp):**
Cholesterol: 0mg
Sodium: 0mg

ALMOND AND COCONUT **butter blend (1 tbsp):**
Cholesterol: 0mg
Sodium: 0mg

HAZELNUT AND FLAXSEED **butter blend (1 tbsp):**
Cholesterol: 0mg
Sodium: 0mg

ALMOND AND CHIA **seed butter blend (1 tbsp):**
Cholesterol: 0mg
Sodium: 0mg

CASHEW AND FLAXSEED **butter blend (1 tbsp):**
Cholesterol: 0mg
Sodium: 0mg

WALNUT AND CHIA **seed butter blend (1 tbsp):**
Cholesterol: 0mg
Sodium: 0mg

PECAN **and almond butter blend (1 tbsp):**
Cholesterol: 0mg
Sodium: 0mg

. . .

SUNFLOWER AND PUMPKIN **seed butter blend (1 tbsp):**
    Cholesterol: 0mg
    Sodium: 0mg

SESAME AND FLAXSEED **butter blend (1 tbsp):**
    Cholesterol: 0mg
    Sodium: 0mg

PEANUT **and almond butter blend (1 tbsp):**
    Cholesterol: 0mg
    Sodium: 0mg

SUNFLOWER AND CHIA **seed butter blend (1 tbsp):**
    Cholesterol: 0mg
    Sodium: 0mg

ALMOND **and sesame seed butter blend (1 tbsp):**
    Cholesterol: 0mg
    Sodium: 0mg

MACADAMIA NUT **and coconut butter blend (1 tbsp):**
    Cholesterol: 0mg
    Sodium: 0mg

PEANUT AND SUNFLOWER **seed butter blend (1 tbsp):**

Cholesterol: 0mg
Sodium: 0mg

Peanut and flaxseed butter blend (1 tbsp):
Cholesterol: 0mg
Sodium: 0mg

Almond and pumpkin seed butter blend (1 tbsp):
Cholesterol: 0mg
Sodium: 0mg

Cashew and pumpkin seed butter blend (1 tbsp):
Cholesterol: 0mg
Sodium: 0mg

Almond and hemp seed butter blend (1 tbsp):
Cholesterol: 0mg
Sodium: 0mg

Unsweetened Nut Milk

Unsweetened Almond Milk (1 cup):
Cholesterol: 0mg
Sodium: 150mg

Unsweetened Cashew Milk (1 cup):
Cholesterol: 0mg
Sodium: 150mg

. . .

UNSWEETENED HAZELNUT MILK (I CUP):
   Cholesterol: 0mg
   Sodium: 160mg

UNSWEETENED MACADAMIA MILK (I CUP):
   Cholesterol: 0mg
   Sodium: 45mg

UNSWEETENED PECAN MILK (I CUP):
   Cholesterol: 0mg
   Sodium: 105mg

UNSWEETENED WALNUT MILK (I CUP):
   Cholesterol: 0mg
   Sodium: 140mg

UNSWEETENED PISTACHIO MILK (I CUP):
   Cholesterol: 0mg
   Sodium: 110mg

UNSWEETENED BRAZIL NUT Milk (I cup):
   Cholesterol: 0mg
   Sodium: 65mg

UNSWEETENED COCONUT MILK (I CUP):

Cholesterol: 0mg
Sodium: 20mg

UNSWEETENED SESAME MILK (1 CUP):
Cholesterol: 0mg
Sodium: 60mg

UNSWEETENED HEMP MILK (1 CUP):
Cholesterol: 0mg
Sodium: 130mg

UNSWEETENED FLAX MILK (1 CUP):
Cholesterol: 0mg
Sodium: 100mg

UNSWEETENED SUNFLOWER MILK (1 CUP):
Cholesterol: 0mg
Sodium: 110mg

UNSWEETENED CHIA MILK (1 CUP):
Cholesterol: 0mg
Sodium: 10mg

UNSWEETENED PINE NUT MILK (1 cup):
Cholesterol: 0mg
Sodium: 5mg

. . .

UNSWEETENED OAT MILK (1 CUP):
  Cholesterol: 0mg
  Sodium: 100mg

UNSWEETENED RICE MILK (1 CUP):
  Cholesterol: 0mg
  Sodium: 120mg

UNSWEETENED QUINOA MILK (1 CUP):
  Cholesterol: 0mg
  Sodium: 150mg

UNSWEETENED PEA MILK (1 CUP):
  Cholesterol: 0mg
  Sodium: 150mg

UNSWEETENED SOY MILK (1 CUP):
  Cholesterol: 0mg
  Sodium: 80mg

UNSWEETENED BLACK SESAME Milk (1 cup):
  Cholesterol: 0mg
  Sodium: 5mg

UNSWEETENED CHESTNUT MILK (1 CUP):
  Cholesterol: 0mg
  Sodium: 5mg

. . .

UNSWEETENED PUMPKIN SEED Milk (1 cup):
    Cholesterol: 0mg
    Sodium: 150mg

UNSWEETENED POPPY SEED Milk (1 cup):
    Cholesterol: 0mg
    Sodium: 60mg

UNSWEETENED AMARANTH MILK (1 CUP):
    Cholesterol: 0mg
    Sodium: 5mg

UNSWEETENED MORINGA SEED Milk (1 cup):
    Cholesterol: 0mg
    Sodium: 150mg

UNSWEETENED WATERMELON SEED Milk (1 cup):
    Cholesterol: 0mg
    Sodium: 150mg

UNSWEETENED ALMOND-CASHEW MILK Blend (1 cup):
    Cholesterol: 0mg
    Sodium: 150mg

UNSWEETENED ALMOND-COCONUT MILK Blend (1 cup):

Cholesterol: 0mg
Sodium: 170mg

UNSWEETENED CASHEW-COCONUT MILK **Blend (1 cup):**
Cholesterol: 0mg
Sodium: 150mg

UNSWEETENED MACADAMIA-COCONUT MILK **Blend (1 cup):**
Cholesterol: 0mg
Sodium: 40mg

UNSWEETENED HAZELNUT-CASHEW MILK **Blend (1 cup):**
Cholesterol: 0mg
Sodium: 110mg

UNSWEETENED WALNUT-PECAN MILK **Blend (1 cup):**
Cholesterol: 0mg
Sodium: 90mg

UNSWEETENED ALMOND-HEMP MILK **Blend (1 cup):**
Cholesterol: 0mg
Sodium: 180mg

UNSWEETENED ALMOND-FLAX MILK **Blend (1 cup):**
Cholesterol: 0mg
Sodium: 150mg

. . .

UNSWEETENED CASHEW-SESAME MILK Blend (1 cup):
 Cholesterol: 0mg
 Sodium: 70mg

UNSWEETENED ALMOND-OAT MILK Blend (1 cup):
 Cholesterol: 0mg
 Sodium: 100mg

UNSWEETENED ALMOND-RICE MILK Blend (1 cup):
 Cholesterol: 0mg
 Sodium: 150mg

UNSWEETENED HAZELNUT-SOY MILK Blend (1 cup):
 Cholesterol: 0mg
 Sodium: 80mg

UNSWEETENED ALMOND-PEA MILK Blend (1 cup):
 Cholesterol: 0mg
 Sodium: 150mg

UNSWEETENED ALMOND-SUNFLOWER MILK Blend (1 cup):
 Cholesterol: 0mg
 Sodium: 160mg

UNSWEETENED ALMOND-QUINOA MILK Blend (1 cup):
 Cholesterol: 0mg
 Sodium: 160mg

. . .

UNSWEETENED ALMOND-PISTACHIO MILK Blend (1 cup):
Cholesterol: 0mg
Sodium: 120mg

UNSWEETENED ALMOND-BLACK SESAME Milk Blend (1 cup):
Cholesterol: 0mg
Sodium: 5mg

UNSWEETENED ALMOND-PUMPKIN SEED Milk Blend (1 cup):
Cholesterol: 0mg
Sodium: 150mg

UNSWEETENED ALMOND-POPPY SEED Milk Blend (1 cup):
Cholesterol: 0mg
Sodium: 70mg

UNSWEETENED CASHEW-HEMP MILK Blend (1 cup):
Cholesterol: 0mg
Sodium: 180mg

UNSWEETENED CASHEW-FLAX MILK Blend (1 cup):
Cholesterol: 0mg
Sodium: 150mg

UNSWEETENED CASHEW-SESAME MILK Blend (1 cup):

Cholesterol: 0mg
Sodium: 70mg

UNSWEETENED MACADAMIA-SOY MILK Blend (1 cup):
Cholesterol: 0mg
Sodium: 80mg

Dairy and dairy alternatives:

Low-fat or Fat-free Milk

Skim Milk:
Cholesterol: 2mg
Sodium: 126mg

FAT-FREE MILK:
Cholesterol: 2mg
Sodium: 130mg

1% Milk:
Cholesterol: 5mg
Sodium: 107mg

2% Reduced Fat Milk:
Cholesterol: 20mg
Sodium: 122mg

· · ·

Semi-Skimmed Milk:
Cholesterol: 8mg
Sodium: 120mg

Low-Fat Dairy Milk:
Cholesterol: 8mg
Sodium: 120mg

Light Milk:
Cholesterol: 5mg
Sodium: 120mg

Slim Milk:
Cholesterol: 2mg
Sodium: 126mg

Part-Skim Milk:
Cholesterol: 20mg
Sodium: 124mg

1% Reduced Milk:
Cholesterol: 5mg
Sodium: 107mg

Ultra-Low-Fat Milk:
Cholesterol: 2mg
Sodium: 125mg

. . .

Non-Fat Milk:
Cholesterol: 2mg
Sodium: 130mg

Fat-Trimmed Milk:
Cholesterol: 5mg
Sodium: 120mg

Low-Calorie Milk:
Cholesterol: 2mg
Sodium: 126mg

Reduced-Fat Dairy Milk:
Cholesterol: 20mg
Sodium: 120mg

Skinny Milk:
Cholesterol: 2mg
Sodium: 126mg

Trim Milk:
Cholesterol: 2mg
Sodium: 126mg

Lightly Skimmed Milk:

Cholesterol: 8mg
Sodium: 120mg

0.5% Milk:
Cholesterol: 8mg
Sodium: 120mg

Low-Fat Cow's Milk:
Cholesterol: 5mg
Sodium: 120mg

Half-Skimmed Milk:
Cholesterol: 8mg
Sodium: 120mg

98% Fat-Free Milk:
Cholesterol: 5mg
Sodium: 120mg

1/2% Milk:
Cholesterol: 8mg
Sodium: 120mg

Diet Milk:
Cholesterol: 2mg
Sodium: 126mg

. . .

Lite Milk:
　　Cholesterol: 2mg
　　Sodium: 130mg

Low-Fat Lactose-Free Milk:
　　Cholesterol: 2mg
　　Sodium: 130mg

Slimmed Milk:
　　Cholesterol: 5mg
　　Sodium: 120mg

Skimmed Dairy Milk:
　　Cholesterol: 2mg
　　Sodium: 126mg

99% Fat-Free Milk:
　　Cholesterol: 2mg
　　Sodium: 130mg

1/3% Milk:
　　Cholesterol: 8mg
　　Sodium: 120mg

Lean Milk:
　　Cholesterol: 8mg
　　Sodium: 120mg

. . .

Half Percent Milk:
Cholesterol: 8mg
Sodium: 120mg

1/4% Milk:
Cholesterol: 8mg
Sodium: 120mg

Reduced Lactose Milk:
Cholesterol: 2mg
Sodium: 125mg

Low-Fat Homogenized Milk:
Cholesterol: 8mg
Sodium: 120mg

Lightly Fat-Free Milk:
Cholesterol: 2mg
Sodium: 126mg

Low-Fat Pasteurized Milk:
Cholesterol: 8mg
Sodium: 120mg

0.1% Milk:

Cholesterol: 8mg
Sodium: 120mg

DIETETIC MILK:
Cholesterol: 2mg
Sodium: 126mg

SUPER SKIM MILK:
Cholesterol: 2mg
Sodium: 130mg

LACTOSE-REDUCED MILK:
Cholesterol: 2mg
Sodium: 130mg

LOW-FAT ULTRA-PASTEURIZED MILK:
Cholesterol: 8mg
Sodium: 120mg

EXTRA LIGHT MILK:
Cholesterol: 2mg
Sodium: 126mg

LOW-FAT UHT MILK:
Cholesterol: 2mg
Sodium: 130mg

. . .

1/8% Milk:
　　Cholesterol: 8mg
　　Sodium: 120mg

CALORIE-CONSCIOUS MILK:
　　Cholesterol: 2mg
　　Sodium: 126mg

LOW-FAT FRESH MILK:
　　Cholesterol: 2mg
　　Sodium: 126mg

LOW-FAT ASEPTIC MILK:
　　Cholesterol: 2mg
　　Sodium: 126mg

LOW-FAT ORGANIC MILK:
　　Cholesterol: 2mg
　　Sodium: 126mg

0.2% Milk:
　　Cholesterol: 8mg
　　Sodium: 120mg

YOGURT (1 CUP SERVING):
　　Cholesterol: 10mg
　　Sodium: 150mg

. . .

Cottage Cheese (1/2 cup serving):
Cholesterol: 5mg
Sodium: 350mg

Reduced-fat Cheese

Reduced-Fat Cheddar:
Cholesterol: 6mg
Sodium: 174mg

Low-Fat Mozzarella:
Cholesterol: 8mg
Sodium: 176mg

Part-Skim Ricotta:
Cholesterol: 14mg
Sodium: 46mg

Light Swiss Cheese:
Cholesterol: 9mg
Sodium: 45mg

Reduced-Fat Gouda:
Cholesterol: 8mg
Sodium: 217mg

. . .

2% Milk Pepper Jack:
Cholesterol: 7mg
Sodium: 170mg

Half-Fat Colby:
Cholesterol: 12mg
Sodium: 184mg

Semi-Skimmed Monterey Jack:
Cholesterol: 12mg
Sodium: 178mg

Low-Fat Havarti:
Cholesterol: 11mg
Sodium: 198mg

1% Milk Provolone:
Cholesterol: 5mg
Sodium: 220mg

Skim Milk Gruyere:
Cholesterol: 5mg
Sodium: 55mg

Lite Blue Cheese:
Cholesterol: 8mg
Sodium: 240mg

. . .

2% Milk Brie:
    Cholesterol: 12mg
    Sodium: 178mg

Part-Skim Feta:
    Cholesterol: 16mg
    Sodium: 316mg

Low-Fat Parmesan:
    Cholesterol: 7mg
    Sodium: 152mg

Light Gorgonzola:
    Cholesterol: 5mg
    Sodium: 192mg

1% Milk Gouda:
    Cholesterol: 9mg
    Sodium: 185mg

Half-Fat Camembert:
    Cholesterol: 25mg
    Sodium: 272mg

Semi-Skimmed Fontina:

Cholesterol: 9mg
Sodium: 142mg

Low-Fat Gouda:
Cholesterol: 10mg
Sodium: 200mg

Lite Gruyere:
Cholesterol: 12mg
Sodium: 50mg

2% Milk Edam:
Cholesterol: 7mg
Sodium: 187mg

Part-Skim Muenster:
Cholesterol: 13mg
Sodium: 165mg

Reduced-Fat Havarti:
Cholesterol: 11mg
Sodium: 195mg

Light Monterey Jack:
Cholesterol: 9mg
Sodium: 160mg

. . .

SKIM MILK BOURSAULT:
    Cholesterol: 11mg
    Sodium: 350mg

LOW-FAT CAMEMBERT:
    Cholesterol: 20mg
    Sodium: 258mg

1% Milk Roquefort:
    Cholesterol: 17mg
    Sodium: 498mg

HALF-FAT GOUDA:
    Cholesterol: 7mg
    Sodium: 210mg

SEMI-SKIMMED PROVOLONE:
    Cholesterol: 8mg
    Sodium: 243mg

LOW-FAT BLUE CHEESE:
    Cholesterol: 8mg
    Sodium: 204mg

LITE EMMENTAL:
    Cholesterol: 10mg
    Sodium: 54mg

. . .

2% Milk Romano:
   Cholesterol: 6mg
   Sodium: 360mg

PART-SKIM GOUDA:
   Cholesterol: 9mg
   Sodium: 220mg

REDUCED-FAT COLBY:
   Cholesterol: 15mg
   Sodium: 188mg

LIGHT JARLSBERG:
   Cholesterol: 10mg
   Sodium: 200mg

SKIM MILK MOZZARELLA:
   Cholesterol: 3mg
   Sodium: 181mg

LOW-FAT PROVOLONE:
   Cholesterol: 7mg
   Sodium: 198mg

1% Milk Cheddar:

Cholesterol: 8mg
Sodium: 174mg

HALF-FAT PARMESAN:
Cholesterol: 9mg
Sodium: 262mg

SEMI-SKIMMED GOUDA:
Cholesterol: 9mg
Sodium: 218mg

Low-Fat Emmental:
Cholesterol: 10mg
Sodium: 56mg

LITE FONTINA:
Cholesterol: 8mg
Sodium: 140mg

2% Milk Havarti:
Cholesterol: 11mg
Sodium: 187mg

PART-SKIM CAMEMBERT:
Cholesterol: 27mg
Sodium: 233mg

. . .

REDUCED-FAT FETA:
>Cholesterol: 17mg
>Sodium: 356mg

LIGHT ROQUEFORT:
>Cholesterol: 9mg
>Sodium: 484mg

Plant-based Milk Alternatives

Skim Milk Swiss:
>Cholesterol: 5mg
>Sodium: 53mg

LOW-FAT GORGONZOLA:
>Cholesterol: 10mg
>Sodium: 189mg

ALMOND MILK:
>Cholesterol: 0mg
>Sodium: 150mg

SOY MILK:
>Cholesterol: 0mg
>Sodium: 80mg

OAT MILK:
>Cholesterol: 0mg

Sodium: 100mg

COCONUT MILK:
Cholesterol: 0mg
Sodium: 15mg

RICE MILK:
Cholesterol: 0mg
Sodium: 120mg

CASHEW MILK:
Cholesterol: 0mg
Sodium: 140mg

HEMP MILK:
Cholesterol: 0mg
Sodium: 100mg

FLAX MILK:
Cholesterol: 0mg
Sodium: 160mg

MACADAMIA MILK:
Cholesterol: 0mg
Sodium: 50mg

. . .

PEA MILK:
    Cholesterol: 0mg
    Sodium: 70mg

WALNUT MILK:
    Cholesterol: 0mg
    Sodium: 135mg

HAZELNUT MILK:
    Cholesterol: 0mg
    Sodium: 110mg

PISTACHIO MILK:
    Cholesterol: 0mg
    Sodium: 80mg

SUNFLOWER SEED MILK:
    Cholesterol: 0mg
    Sodium: 130mg

SESAME MILK:
    Cholesterol: 0mg
    Sodium: 110mg

PECAN MILK:
    Cholesterol: 0mg
    Sodium: 10mg

. . .

Quinoa Milk:
Cholesterol: 0mg
Sodium: 70mg

Chia Milk:
Cholesterol: 0mg
Sodium: 120mg

Pine Nut Milk:
Cholesterol: 0mg
Sodium: 35mg

Brazil Nut Milk:
Cholesterol: 0mg
Sodium: 10mg

Buckwheat Milk:
Cholesterol: 0mg
Sodium: 50mg

Chestnut Milk:
Cholesterol: 0mg
Sodium: 50mg

Spelt Milk:

Cholesterol: 0mg
Sodium: 105mg

HEMP AND RICE BLEND MILK:
Cholesterol: 0mg
Sodium: 130mg

PUMPKIN SEED MILK:
Cholesterol: 0mg
Sodium: 130mg

BARLEY MILK:
Cholesterol: 0mg
Sodium: 80mg

MILLET MILK:
Cholesterol: 0mg
Sodium: 85mg

CASHEW AND ALMOND BLEND MILK:
Cholesterol: 0mg
Sodium: 90mg

FLAX AND OAT BLEND MILK:
Cholesterol: 0mg
Sodium: 110mg

. . .

Pea and Oat Blend Milk:
   Cholesterol: 0mg
   Sodium: 90mg

Coconut and Almond Blend Milk:
   Cholesterol: 0mg
   Sodium: 100mg

Almond and Cashew Blend Milk:
   Cholesterol: 0mg
   Sodium: 110mg

Hazelnut and Oat Blend Milk:
   Cholesterol: 0mg
   Sodium: 90mg

Soy and Rice Blend Milk:
   Cholesterol: 0mg
   Sodium: 100mg

Oat and Rice Blend Milk:
   Cholesterol: 0mg
   Sodium: 80mg

Macadamia and Cashew Blend Milk:
   Cholesterol: 0mg
   Sodium: 70mg

. . .

QUINOA AND RICE BLEND MILK:
    Cholesterol: 0mg
    Sodium: 70mg

SUNFLOWER SEED and Pumpkin Seed Blend Milk:
    Cholesterol: 0mg
    Sodium: 125mg

ALMOND AND COCONUT BLEND MILK:
    Cholesterol: 0mg
    Sodium: 180mg

PECAN AND WALNUT BLEND MILK:
    Cholesterol: 0mg
    Sodium: 15mg

FLAX AND HEMP BLEND MILK:
    Cholesterol: 0mg
    Sodium: 160mg

COCONUT AND RICE BLEND MILK:
    Cholesterol: 0mg
    Sodium: 35mg

ALMOND AND HEMP BLEND MILK:

Cholesterol: 0mg
Sodium: 180mg

CHIA AND OAT BLEND MILK:
Cholesterol: 0mg
Sodium: 100mg

CASHEW AND OAT BLEND MILK:
Cholesterol: 0mg
Sodium: 90mg

COCONUT AND SOY BLEND MILK:
Cholesterol: 0mg
Sodium: 60mg

RICE AND HEMP BLEND MILK:
Cholesterol: 0mg
Sodium: 110mg

ALMOND AND FLAX BLEND MILK:
Cholesterol: 0mg
Sodium: 150mg

HAZELNUT AND RICE BLEND MILK:
Cholesterol: 0mg
Sodium: 110mg

Herbs, spices, and flavor enhancers:

Garlic (1 clove):
Cholesterol: 0mg
Sodium: 1mg

GINGER (1 TSP GRATED):
Cholesterol: 0mg
Sodium: 0mg

TURMERIC (1 TSP):
Cholesterol: 0mg
Sodium: 1mg

CINNAMON (1 TSP):
Cholesterol: 0mg
Sodium: 0mg

BLACK PEPPER (1 TSP):
Cholesterol: 0mg
Sodium: 1mg

BASIL (1 TBSP FRESH):
Cholesterol: 0mg
Sodium: 0mg

OREGANO (1 TBSP FRESH):

Cholesterol: 0mg
Sodium: 0mg

ROSEMARY (1 TBSP FRESH):
Cholesterol: 0mg
Sodium: 1mg

THYME (1 TSP DRIED):
Cholesterol: 0mg
Sodium: 1mg

PAPRIKA (1 TSP):
Cholesterol: 0mg
Sodium: 1mg

CARDAMOM (1 TSP GROUND):
Cholesterol: 0mg
Sodium: 0mg

CLOVES (1 TSP GROUND):
Cholesterol: 0mg
Sodium: 1mg

NUTMEG (1 TSP GROUND):
Cholesterol: 0mg
Sodium: 0mg

. . .

CUMIN (1 TSP GROUND):
    Cholesterol: 0mg
    Sodium: 1mg

CORIANDER (1 TBSP FRESH):
    Cholesterol: 0mg
    Sodium: 1mg

BAY LEAVES (1 LEAF):
    Cholesterol: 0mg
    Sodium: 1mg

SAGE (1 TBSP FRESH):
    Cholesterol: 0mg
    Sodium: 0mg

FENNEL SEEDS (1 TSP):
    Cholesterol: 0mg
    Sodium: 0mg

MUSTARD SEEDS (1 TSP):
    Cholesterol: 0mg
    Sodium: 0mg

ALLSPICE (1 TSP GROUND):
    Cholesterol: 0mg
    Sodium: 1mg

. . .

CHILI POWDER (I TSP):
  Cholesterol: omg
  Sodium: img

DILL (I TBSP FRESH):
  Cholesterol: omg
  Sodium: img

MARJORAM (I TBSP FRESH):
  Cholesterol: omg
  Sodium: omg

SAFFRON (I TSP):
  Cholesterol: omg
  Sodium: omg

PARSLEY (I TBSP FRESH):
  Cholesterol: omg
  Sodium: omg

TARRAGON (I TBSP FRESH):
  Cholesterol: omg
  Sodium: img

MINT (I TBSP FRESH):

Cholesterol: 0mg
Sodium: 1mg

CARAWAY SEEDS (1 TSP):
Cholesterol: 0mg
Sodium: 1mg

ANISE SEEDS (1 TSP):
Cholesterol: 0mg
Sodium: 1mg

FENUGREEK (1 TSP):
Cholesterol: 0mg
Sodium: 2mg

CURRY POWDER (1 TSP):
Cholesterol: 0mg
Sodium: 2mg

CELERY SEEDS (1 TSP):
Cholesterol: 0mg
Sodium: 1mg

JUNIPER BERRIES (1 BERRY):
Cholesterol: 0mg
Sodium: 0mg

. . .

Lemon balm (1 tbsp fresh):
 Cholesterol: 0mg
 Sodium: 1mg

Carom seeds (Ajwain) (1 tsp):
 Cholesterol: 0mg
 Sodium: 1mg

Asafoetida (Hing) (1 tsp):
 Cholesterol: 0mg
 Sodium: 1mg

Vanilla (1 tsp extract):
 Cholesterol: 0mg
 Sodium: 1mg

Mace (1 tsp ground):
 Cholesterol: 0mg
 Sodium: 0mg

Star anise (1 pod):
 Cholesterol: 0mg
 Sodium: 1mg

Peppermint (1 tbsp fresh):
 Cholesterol: 0mg
 Sodium: 0mg

. . .

LEMONGRASS (1 STALK):
Cholesterol: 0mg
Sodium: 0mg

SZECHUAN PEPPER (1 TSP):
Cholesterol: 0mg
Sodium: 0mg

LAVENDER (1 TSP):
Cholesterol: 0mg
Sodium: 0mg

SAVORY (1 TBSP FRESH):
Cholesterol: 0mg
Sodium: 1mg

TAMARIND (1 TBSP PULP):
Cholesterol: 0mg
Sodium: 2mg

LEMON VERBENA (1 TBSP FRESH):
Cholesterol: 0mg
Sodium: 1mg

CILANTRO (CORIANDER LEAVES) (1 tbsp fresh):

Cholesterol: 0mg
Sodium: 1mg

CHIVES (1 TBSP FRESH):
Cholesterol: 0mg
Sodium: 0mg

CURRY LEAVES (1 SPRIG):
Cholesterol: 0mg
Sodium: 1mg

EPAZOTE (1 TBSP FRESH):
Cholesterol: 0mg
Sodium: 1mg

LOVAGE (1 TBSP FRESH):
Cholesterol: 0mg
Sodium: 1mg

LEMON THYME (1 TBSP FRESH):
Cholesterol: 0mg
Sodium: 1mg

LEMON BASIL (1 TBSP FRESH):
Cholesterol: 0mg
Sodium: 1mg

. . .

LEMON PEPPER SEASONING (1 TSP):
    Cholesterol: 0mg
    Sodium: 1mg

LEMON MYRTLE (1 TSP):
    Cholesterol: 0mg
    Sodium: 1mg

LEMON ZEST (1 TSP):
    Cholesterol: 0mg
    Sodium: 0mg

LIME ZEST (1 TSP):
    Cholesterol: 0mg
    Sodium: 0mg

LIME LEAVES (1 LEAF):
    Cholesterol: 0mg
    Sodium: 1mg

BAY LAUREL LEAVES (1 LEAF):
    Cholesterol: 0mg
    Sodium: 0mg

JUNIPER BERRIES (1 BERRY):
    Cholesterol: 0mg
    Sodium: 0mg

. . .

PINK PEPPERCORNS (1 TSP):
    Cholesterol: 0mg
    Sodium: 0mg

WHITE PEPPERCORNS (1 TSP):
    Cholesterol: 0mg
    Sodium: 1mg

GRAINS OF PARADISE (1 TSP):
    Cholesterol: 0mg
    Sodium: 0mg

SUMAC (1 TSP):
    Cholesterol: 0mg
    Sodium: 1mg

ALEPPO PEPPER (1 TSP):
    Cholesterol: 0mg
    Sodium: 1mg

ASAFETIDA (ASAFOETIDA) (1 TSP):
    Cholesterol: 0mg
    Sodium: 0mg

CILANTRO SEEDS (1 TSP):

Cholesterol: 0mg
Sodium: 1mg

NIGELLA SEEDS (1 TSP):
Cholesterol: 0mg
Sodium: 1mg

AJWAIN (CAROM SEEDS) (1 TSP):
Cholesterol: 0mg
Sodium: 0mg

CASSIA BARK (1 INCH PIECE):
Cholesterol: 0mg
Sodium: 1mg

ANNATTO SEEDS (1 TSP):
Cholesterol: 0mg
Sodium: 1mg

ACHIOTE SEEDS (1 TSP):
Cholesterol: 0mg
Sodium: 1mg

CHERVIL (1 TBSP FRESH):
Cholesterol: 0mg
Sodium: 0mg

. . .

LEMON THYME (1 TBSP FRESH):
Cholesterol: 0mg
Sodium: 1mg

LEMON BALM (1 TBSP FRESH):
Cholesterol: 0mg
Sodium: 1mg

LEMON BASIL (1 TBSP FRESH):
Cholesterol: 0mg
Sodium: 1mg

LEMON MYRTLE (1 TSP):
Cholesterol: 0mg
Sodium: 1mg

LEMON ZEST (1 TSP):
Cholesterol: 0mg
Sodium: 0mg

LIME ZEST (1 TSP):
Cholesterol: 0mg
Sodium: 0mg

LIME LEAVES (1 LEAF):
Cholesterol: 0mg
Sodium: 1mg

. . .

BAY LAUREL LEAVES (I LEAF):
  Cholesterol: 0mg
  Sodium: 0mg

JUNIPER BERRIES (I BERRY):
  Cholesterol: 0mg
  Sodium: 0mg

PINK PEPPERCORNS (I TSP):
  Cholesterol: 0mg
  Sodium: 0mg

WHITE PEPPERCORNS (I TSP):
  Cholesterol: 0mg
  Sodium: 1mg

HIGH CHOLESTEROL FOODS TO AVOID

Saturated fat-rich meats:

Red Meats

Beef (lean cuts, cooked, 3 oz serving):
Cholesterol: 70mg
Sodium: 62mg

Lamb (cooked, 3 oz serving):
Cholesterol: 78mg
Sodium: 54mg

Pork (lean cuts, cooked, 3 oz serving):
Cholesterol: 71mg
Sodium: 63mg

Venison (cooked, 3 oz serving):
Cholesterol: 112mg

Sodium: 66mg

Bison (cooked, 3 oz serving):
Cholesterol: 82mg
Sodium: 55mg

Veal (cooked, 3 oz serving):
Cholesterol: 97mg
Sodium: 67mg

Elk (cooked, 3 oz serving):
Cholesterol: 66mg
Sodium: 53mg

Wild Boar (cooked, 3 oz serving):
Cholesterol: 60mg
Sodium: 59mg

Kangaroo (cooked, 3 oz serving):
Cholesterol: 60mg
Sodium: 53mg

Ostrich (cooked, 3 oz serving):
Cholesterol: 57mg
Sodium: 68mg

Goat (cooked, 3 oz serving):
Cholesterol: 63mg
Sodium: 67mg

Rabbit (cooked, 3 oz serving):
Cholesterol: 109mg
Sodium: 49mg

Horse (cooked, 3 oz serving):
Cholesterol: 53mg
Sodium: 62mg

Antelope (cooked, 3 oz serving):
Cholesterol: 114mg
Sodium: 63mg

Llama (cooked, 3 oz serving):
Cholesterol: 56mg
Sodium: 45mg

Caribou (cooked, 3 oz serving):
Cholesterol: 74mg
Sodium: 64mg

Camel (cooked, 3 oz serving):
Cholesterol: 85mg
Sodium: 60mg

Guinea Pig (cooked, 3 oz serving):
Cholesterol: 55mg
Sodium: 44mg

Alligator (cooked, 3 oz serving):
Cholesterol: 60mg
Sodium: 57mg

Emu (cooked, 3 oz serving):
Cholesterol: 64mg
Sodium: 51mg

Grouse (cooked, 3 oz serving):
Cholesterol: 142mg
Sodium: 53mg

Moose (cooked, 3 oz serving):
Cholesterol: 73mg
Sodium: 60mg

Quail (cooked, 3 oz serving):
Cholesterol: 74mg
Sodium: 60mg

Turtle (cooked, 3 oz serving):
Cholesterol: 50mg
Sodium: 70mg

Wild Duck (cooked, 3 oz serving):
Cholesterol: 86mg
Sodium: 57mg

Pheasant (cooked, 3 oz serving):
Cholesterol: 172mg
Sodium: 59mg

Reindeer (cooked, 3 oz serving):
Cholesterol: 83mg
Sodium: 56mg

Bear (cooked, 3 oz serving):
Cholesterol: 82mg
Sodium: 51mg

Wild Turkey (cooked, 3 oz serving):

Cholesterol: 58mg
Sodium: 70mg

Rattlesnake (cooked, 3 oz serving):
Cholesterol: 49mg
Sodium: 42mg

Hare (cooked, 3 oz serving):
Cholesterol: 129mg
Sodium: 65mg

Yak (cooked, 3 oz serving):
Cholesterol: 64mg
Sodium: 53mg

Musk Ox (cooked, 3 oz serving):
Cholesterol: 70mg
Sodium: 53mg

Wallaby (cooked, 3 oz serving):
Cholesterol: 75mg
Sodium: 60mg

Wapiti (Elk meat, cooked, 3 oz serving):
Cholesterol: 55mg
Sodium: 58mg

Boar (cooked, 3 oz serving):
Cholesterol: 82mg
Sodium: 55mg

Muskrat (cooked, 3 oz serving):
Cholesterol: 102mg

Sodium: 62mg

Water Buffalo (cooked, 3 oz serving):
Cholesterol: 71mg
Sodium: 65mg

Haggis (cooked, 3 oz serving):
Cholesterol: 81mg
Sodium: 590mg

Koala (cooked, 3 oz serving):
Cholesterol: 50mg
Sodium: 60mg

Hedgehog (cooked, 3 oz serving):
Cholesterol: 68mg
Sodium: 75mg

Squirrel (cooked, 3 oz serving):
Cholesterol: 68mg
Sodium: 75mg

Nutria (Coypu, cooked, 3 oz serving):
Cholesterol: 75mg
Sodium: 65mg

Zebra (cooked, 3 oz serving):
Cholesterol: 98mg
Sodium: 66mg

Armadillo (cooked, 3 oz serving):
Cholesterol: 60mg
Sodium: 70mg

Porcupine (cooked, 3 oz serving):
Cholesterol: 65mg
Sodium: 40mg

Snapping Turtle (cooked, 3 oz serving):
Cholesterol: 56mg
Sodium: 70mg

Puffin (cooked, 3 oz serving):
Cholesterol: 50mg
Sodium: 90mg

Weasel (cooked, 3 oz serving):
Cholesterol: 82mg
Sodium: 76mg

Chipmunk (cooked, 3 oz serving):
Cholesterol: 78mg
Sodium: 68mg

Skunk (cooked, 3 oz serving):
Cholesterol: 54mg
Sodium: 60mg

Raccoon (cooked, 3 oz serving):
Cholesterol: 76mg
Sodium: 76mg

Marmot (cooked, 3 oz serving):
Cholesterol: 76mg
Sodium: 76mg

Wild Sheep (cooked, 3 oz serving):
Cholesterol: 73mg
Sodium: 61mg

Wild Goat (cooked, 3 oz serving):
Cholesterol: 82mg
Sodium: 55mg

Wallaroo (cooked, 3 oz serving):
Cholesterol: 85mg
Sodium: 57mg

Organ Meats

Beef Liver (3 oz serving):
Cholesterol: 331mg
Sodium: 89mg

Beef Kidneys (3 oz serving):
Cholesterol: 332mg
Sodium: 94mg

Beef Heart (3 oz serving):
Cholesterol: 129mg
Sodium: 74mg

Beef Tripe (3 oz serving):
Cholesterol: 77mg
Sodium: 80mg

Beef Sweetbreads (Thymus glands) (3 oz serving):
Cholesterol: 123mg

Sodium: 165mg

Beef Tongue (3 oz serving):
Cholesterol: 77mg
Sodium: 73mg

Beef Spleen (3 oz serving):
Cholesterol: 258mg
Sodium: 85mg

Beef Brain (3 oz serving):
Cholesterol: 1,033mg
Sodium: 49mg

Beef Oxtail (3 oz serving):
Cholesterol: 92mg
Sodium: 66mg

Beef Cheeks (3 oz serving):
Cholesterol: 96mg
Sodium: 56mg

Chicken Liver (3 oz serving):
Cholesterol: 185mg
Sodium: 69mg

Chicken Hearts (3 oz serving):
Cholesterol: 236mg
Sodium: 74mg

Chicken Gizzards (3 oz serving):
Cholesterol: 180mg
Sodium: 75mg

Chicken Neck (3 oz serving):
Cholesterol: 70mg
Sodium: 68mg

Chicken Feet (3 oz serving):
Cholesterol: 171mg
Sodium: 63mg

Chicken Comb and Wattles (3 oz serving):
Cholesterol: 79mg
Sodium: 90mg

Chicken Testicles (Rooster's) (3 oz serving):
Cholesterol: 364mg
Sodium: 147mg

Chicken Oysters (located on the back) (3 oz serving):
Cholesterol: 177mg
Sodium: 70mg

Chicken Livers (Fried or Grilled) (3 oz serving):
Cholesterol: 271mg
Sodium: 133mg

Pork Liver (3 oz serving):
Cholesterol: 324mg
Sodium: 73mg

Pork Kidneys (3 oz serving):
Cholesterol: 347mg
Sodium: 69mg

Pork Heart (3 oz serving):
Cholesterol: 129mg
Sodium: 65mg

Pork Brain (3 oz serving):
Cholesterol: 1,033mg
Sodium: 33mg

Pork Spleen (3 oz serving):
Cholesterol: 268mg
Sodium: 109mg

Pork Sweetbreads (3 oz serving):
Cholesterol: 181mg
Sodium: 85mg

Pork Tongue (3 oz serving):
Cholesterol: 106mg
Sodium: 51mg

Pork Tripe (Stomach Lining) (3 oz serving):
Cholesterol: 66mg
Sodium: 99mg

Pork Tails (Pig's Tail) (3 oz serving):
Cholesterol: 97mg
Sodium: 63mg

Pork Ears (Pig's Ears) (3 oz serving):
Cholesterol: 73mg
Sodium: 208mg

Lamb Liver (3 oz serving):

Cholesterol: 287mg
Sodium: 64mg

Lamb Kidneys (3 oz serving):
Cholesterol: 332mg
Sodium: 84mg

Lamb Heart (3 oz serving):
Cholesterol: 111mg
Sodium: 64mg

Lamb Sweetbreads (3 oz serving):
Cholesterol: 150mg
Sodium: 66mg

Lamb Tongue (3 oz serving):
Cholesterol: 95mg
Sodium: 50mg

Lamb Tripe (3 oz serving):
Cholesterol: 77mg
Sodium: 74mg

Lamb Brain (3 oz serving):
Cholesterol: 1,033mg
Sodium: 33mg

Lamb Spleen (3 oz serving):
Cholesterol: 389mg
Sodium: 91mg

Lamb Testicles (3 oz serving):
Cholesterol: 290mg

Sodium: 95mg

Lamb Sweetbreads (3 oz serving):
Cholesterol: 150mg
Sodium: 66mg

Beef Tongue Tacos (3 oz serving):
Cholesterol: 77mg
Sodium: 57mg

Pork Brain Fritters (3 oz serving):
Cholesterol: 1,033mg
Sodium: 61mg

Lamb Sweetbreads w/ Mustard Sauce (3 oz serving):
Cholesterol: 150mg
Sodium: 260mg

Chicken Heart Skewers (3 oz serving):
Cholesterol: 236mg
Sodium: 74mg

Pork Cheek Confit (3 oz serving):
Cholesterol: 93mg
Sodium: 83mg

Lamb Tongue Stew (3 oz serving):
Cholesterol: 95mg
Sodium: 56mg

Beef Tripe Soup (Menudo) (3 oz serving):
Cholesterol: 77mg
Sodium: 96mg

Chicken Gizzard Stir-Fry (3 oz serving):
Cholesterol: 180mg
Sodium: 111mg

Pork Kidney Curry (3 oz serving):
Cholesterol: 347mg
Sodium: 94mg

Lamb Brain Masala (3 oz serving):
Cholesterol: 1,033mg
Sodium: 44mg

Mixed Organ Meats Stir-Fry (3 oz serving):
Cholesterol: Varies depending on the mix of organs
Sodium: Varies depending on the mix of organs

Processed Meats

Bacon (3 oz serving):
Cholesterol: 87mg
Sodium: 1,282mg

Salami (3 oz serving):
Cholesterol: 70mg
Sodium: 1,607mg

Hot dogs (3 oz serving):
Cholesterol: 36mg
Sodium: 852mg

Bologna (3 oz serving):

Cholesterol: 33mg
Sodium: 973mg

Pepperoni (3 oz serving):
Cholesterol: 97mg
Sodium: 1,446mg

Ham (3 oz serving):
Cholesterol: 38mg
Sodium: 1,028mg

Prosciutto (3 oz serving):
Cholesterol: 51mg
Sodium: 1,032mg

Mortadella (3 oz serving):
Cholesterol: 40mg
Sodium: 968mg

Sausages (3 oz serving):
Cholesterol: Varies depending on the type of sausage
Sodium: Varies depending on the type of sausage

Corned beef (3 oz serving):
Cholesterol: 70mg
Sodium: 964mg

Pastrami (3 oz serving):
Cholesterol: 95mg
Sodium: 1,327mg

Canadian bacon (3 oz serving):
Cholesterol: 50mg

Sodium: 1,038mg

Turkey bacon (3 oz serving):
Cholesterol: 37mg
Sodium: 901mg

Bratwurst (3 oz serving):
Cholesterol: 64mg
Sodium: 663mg

Chorizo (3 oz serving):
Cholesterol: 77mg
Sodium: 826mg

Andouille sausage (3 oz serving):
Cholesterol: 60mg
Sodium: 1,080mg

Liverwurst (3 oz serving):
Cholesterol: 94mg
Sodium: 950mg

Krakowska sausage (3 oz serving):
Cholesterol: 70mg
Sodium: 672mg

Vienna sausage (3 oz serving):
Cholesterol: 58mg
Sodium: 876mg

Spam (3 oz serving):
Cholesterol: 69mg
Sodium: 767mg

Beef jerky (3 oz serving):
Cholesterol: 50mg
Sodium: 897mg

Capicola (3 oz serving):
Cholesterol: 45mg
Sodium: 1,035mg

Lebanon bologna (3 oz serving):
Cholesterol: 30mg
Sodium: 1,142mg

Pancetta (3 oz serving):
Cholesterol: 39mg
Sodium: 492mg

Summer sausage (3 oz serving):
Cholesterol: 72mg
Sodium: 978mg

Head cheese (3 oz serving):
Cholesterol: 59mg
Sodium: 663mg

Black forest ham (3 oz serving):
Cholesterol: 44mg
Sodium: 1,254mg

Frankfurters (3 oz serving):
Cholesterol: 35mg
Sodium: 1,049mg

Genoa salami (3 oz serving):
Cholesterol: 45mg
Sodium: 1,035mg

Cervelat sausage (3 oz serving):
Cholesterol: 64mg
Sodium: 783mg

Thuringer sausage (3 oz serving):
Cholesterol: 74mg
Sodium: 920mg

Black pudding (3 oz serving):
Cholesterol: 37mg
Sodium: 988mg

Blood sausage (3 oz serving):
Cholesterol: 46mg
Sodium: 719mg

Deviled ham (3 oz serving):
Cholesterol: 40mg
Sodium: 1,170mg

Chicken nuggets (3 oz serving):
Cholesterol: 37mg
Sodium: 494mg

Chicken sausages (3 oz serving):
Cholesterol: Varies on the type of chicken sausage
Sodium: Varies on the type of chicken sausage

Knockwurst (3 oz serving):

Cholesterol: 69mg
Sodium: 1,209mg

Landjäger (3 oz serving):
Cholesterol: 60mg
Sodium: 1,530mg

Italian sausage (3 oz serving):
Cholesterol: 71mg
Sodium: 780mg

Goetta (3 oz serving):
Cholesterol: 55mg
Sodium: 398mg

Peperoncino (3 oz serving):
Cholesterol: 70mg
Sodium: 2,010mg

Snack sticks (3 oz serving):
Cholesterol: Varies on the brand and type of snack stick
Sodium: Varies on the brand and type of snack stick

Mettwurst (3 oz serving):
Cholesterol: 68mg
Sodium: 1,140mg

Presskopf (3 oz serving):
Cholesterol: 69mg
Sodium: 765mg

Kielbasa (3 oz serving):
Cholesterol: 70mg

Sodium: 1,021mg

Liver sausage (3 oz serving):
Cholesterol: 113mg
Sodium: 659mg

Roast beef (deli-style) (3 oz serving):
Cholesterol: 60mg
Sodium: 1,009mg

Taylor ham (pork roll) (3 oz serving):
Cholesterol: 63mg
Sodium: 727mg

Speck (3 oz serving):
Cholesterol: 65mg
Sodium: 1,280mg

Cajun boudin (3 oz serving):
Cholesterol: 65mg
Sodium: 937mg

Merguez sausage (3 oz serving):
Cholesterol: 73mg
Sodium: 1,201mg

Cotecchino (3 oz serving):
Cholesterol: 84mg
Sodium: 705mg

Muffuletta (3 oz serving):
Cholesterol: 43mg
Sodium: 1,173mg

Black forest turkey (3 oz serving):
Cholesterol: 56mg
Sodium: 982mg

German bologna (3 oz serving):
Cholesterol: 54mg
Sodium: 892mg

Liver pâté (3 oz serving):
Cholesterol: 246mg
Sodium: 621mg

Polony (3 oz serving):
Cholesterol: 40mg
Sodium: 860mg

Cabanossi (3 oz serving):
Cholesterol: 57mg
Sodium: 760mg

Morteau sausage (3 oz serving):
Cholesterol: 92mg
Sodium: 1,535mg

Sobrasada (3 oz serving):
Cholesterol: 71mg
Sodium: 1,200mg

Full-fat dairy products:

Whole Milk

Whole milk (1 cup serving):
Cholesterol: 33mg
Sodium: 122mg

Full-fat Yogurt (1 cup serving):
Cholesterol: 31mg
Sodium: 58mg

Butter (1 tablespoon serving):
Cholesterol: 31mg
Sodium: 87mg

Full-fat Cheese (1 oz serving):
Cholesterol: Varies, typically between 20-30mg
Sodium: Varies, typically between 150-300mg

Full-fat Greek Yogurt (1 cup serving):
Cholesterol: 31mg
Sodium: 56mg

Ghee (Clarified Butter) (1 tablespoon serving):
Cholesterol: 33mg
Sodium: 0mg

Brie Cheese (1 oz serving):
Cholesterol: 32mg
Sodium: 178mg

Full-Fat Cheese
Cottage Cheese (Full-fat) (1 cup serving):

Cholesterol: 48mg
Sodium: 918mg

Roquefort Cheese (1 oz serving):
Cholesterol: 32mg
Sodium: 498mg

Cream Cheese (1 oz serving):
Cholesterol: 29mg
Sodium: 80mg

Ricotta Cheese (Full-fat) (1 cup serving):
Cholesterol: 116mg
Sodium: 92mg

Whipped Cream (1 cup serving):
Cholesterol: 88mg
Sodium: 55mg

Havarti Cheese (1 oz serving):
Cholesterol: 30mg
Sodium: 125mg

Double Gloucester Cheese (1 oz serving):
Cholesterol: 30mg
Sodium: 174mg

Stilton Cheese (1 oz serving):
Cholesterol: 33mg
Sodium: 380mg

Beurre d'Isigny (French Butter) (1 tablespoon serving):
Cholesterol: 31mg

Sodium: 0mg

Gouda Cheese (1 oz serving):
Cholesterol: 27mg
Sodium: 192mg

Neufchâtel Cheese (1 oz serving):
Cholesterol: 27mg
Sodium: 119mg

Danish Blue Cheese (1 oz serving):
Cholesterol: 28mg
Sodium: 360mg

Quark Cheese (1 cup serving):
Cholesterol: 97mg
Sodium: 372mg

Lancashire Cheese (1 oz serving):
Cholesterol: 31mg
Sodium: 204mg

Mascarpone Cream Cheese (1 oz serving):
Cholesterol: 29mg
Sodium: 10mg

Limburger Cheese (1 oz serving):
Cholesterol: 30mg
Sodium: 352mg

Skyr (Icelandic Yogurt) (1 cup serving):
Cholesterol: 25mg
Sodium: 100mg

Munster Cheese (1 oz serving):
Cholesterol: 29mg
Sodium: 189mg

Emmental Cheese (1 oz serving):
Cholesterol: 27mg
Sodium: 74mg

Appenzeller Cheese (1 oz serving):
Cholesterol: 24mg
Sodium: 63mg

Feta Cheese (Full-fat) (1 oz serving):
Cholesterol: 25mg
Sodium: 314mg

Gruyère Cheese (1 oz serving):
Cholesterol: 28mg
Sodium: 74mg

Pont-l'Évêque Cheese (1 oz serving):
Cholesterol: 26mg
Sodium: 180mg

Fromage Blanc (1 cup serving):
Cholesterol: 66mg
Sodium: 94mg

Manchego Cheese (1 oz serving):
Cholesterol: 28mg
Sodium: 198mg

Dolcelatte Cheese (1 oz serving):
Cholesterol: 31mg
Sodium: 345mg

Roncal Cheese (1 oz serving):
Cholesterol: 50mg
Sodium: 150mg

Pyrenees Brebis Cheese (1 oz serving):
Cholesterol: 27mg
Sodium: 60mg

Burrata Cheese (1 oz serving):
Cholesterol: 30mg
Sodium: 28mg

Bel Paese Cheese (1 oz serving):
Cholesterol: 22mg
Sodium: 69mg

Cabrales Cheese (1 oz serving):
Cholesterol: 25mg
Sodium: 480mg

Wensleydale Cheese (Full-fat) (1 oz serving):
Cholesterol: 28mg
Sodium: 174mg

Époisses Cheese (1 oz serving):
Cholesterol: 28mg
Sodium: 240mg

Ardrahan Cheese (1 oz serving):

Cholesterol: 26mg
Sodium: 240mg

Casu Marzu (Sardinian Cheese) (1 oz serving):
Cholesterol: 95mg
Sodium: 2mg

Pecorino Romano Cheese (1 oz serving):
Cholesterol: 27mg
Sodium: 406mg

Ossau-Iraty Cheese (1 oz serving):
Cholesterol: 27mg
Sodium: 70mg

Munster-Géromé Cheese (1 oz serving):
Cholesterol: 27mg
Sodium: 200mg

Majorero Cheese (1 oz serving):
Cholesterol: 32mg
Sodium: 135mg

Dobrodar Cheese (1 oz serving):
Cholesterol: 31mg
Sodium: 240mg

Grana Padano Cheese (1 oz serving):
Cholesterol: 30mg
Sodium: 390mg

Livarot Cheese (1 oz serving):
Cholesterol: 25mg

Sodium: 350mg

Tête de Moine Cheese (1 oz serving):
Cholesterol: 30mg
Sodium: 140mg

Fried and processed foods:

Deep-fried Foods

Deep-fried chicken wings (4 wings):
Cholesterol: 70mg
Sodium: 760mg

Fried calamari (1 cup):
Cholesterol: 245mg
Sodium: 605mg

Deep-fried mozzarella sticks (4 pieces):
Cholesterol: 63mg
Sodium: 620mg

Fried shrimp (3 oz serving):
Cholesterol: 179mg
Sodium: 281mg

Fried bacon strips (3 strips):
Cholesterol: 37mg
Sodium: 475mg

Deep-fried cheese curds (1 cup):
Cholesterol: 95mg
Sodium: 1170mg

Fried chicken tenders (3 tenders):
Cholesterol: 46mg
Sodium: 330mg

Deep-fried egg rolls (1 roll):
Cholesterol: 32mg
Sodium: 220mg

Fried catfish (3 oz serving):
Cholesterol: 58mg
Sodium: 643mg

Fried macaroni and cheese bites (1 serving):
Cholesterol: 25mg
Sodium: 310mg

Deep-fried pickles (5 pickles):
Cholesterol: 0mg
Sodium: 1370mg

Fried churros (1 churro):
Cholesterol: 0mg
Sodium: 110mg

Deep-fried sausage rolls (1 roll):
Cholesterol: 24mg
Sodium: 420mg

Fried coconut shrimp (4 shrimp):

Cholesterol: 40mg
Sodium: 560mg

Deep-fried crab cakes (1 cake):
Cholesterol: 95mg
Sodium: 430mg

Fried chicken nuggets (6 pieces):
Cholesterol: 33mg
Sodium: 460mg

Fried chicken livers (3 oz serving):
Cholesterol: 260mg
Sodium: 222mg

Deep-fried corn dogs (1 corn dog):
Cholesterol: 32mg
Sodium: 990mg

Deep-fried Monte Cristo sandwiches (1 sandwich):
Cholesterol: 89mg
Sodium: 1510mg

Fried chicken gizzards (1 cup):
Cholesterol: 536mg
Sodium: 141mg

Deep-fried zucchini sticks (10 sticks):
Cholesterol: 0mg
Sodium: 760mg

Fried cheese fritters (4 fritters):
Cholesterol: 115mg

Sodium: 325mg

Fried pork chops (3 oz serving):
Cholesterol: 63mg
Sodium: 77mg

Fried crawfish tails (1 cup):
Cholesterol: 221mg
Sodium: 322mg

Deep-fried Camembert cheese (1 oz):
Cholesterol: 30mg
Sodium: 180mg

Fried chicken skin (1 oz):
Cholesterol: 90mg
Sodium: 270mg

Deep-fried fish and chips (1 serving):
Cholesterol: 64mg
Sodium: 600mg

Fried cheddar cheese cubes (1 cup):
Cholesterol: 95mg
Sodium: 180mg

Deep-fried haddock (3 oz serving):
Cholesterol: 65mg
Sodium: 332mg

Fried chicken-fried steak (1 steak):
Cholesterol: 123mg
Sodium: 1190mg

Fried chitterlings (pork intestines) (3 oz serving):
Cholesterol: 351mg
Sodium: 240mg

Fried pork chops (3 oz serving):
Cholesterol: 63mg
Sodium: 77mg

Fried cheddar cheese cubes (1 cup):
Cholesterol: 95mg
Sodium: 180mg

Deep-fried Brie (1 oz):
Cholesterol: 26mg
Sodium: 178mg

Deep-fried haddock (3 oz serving):
Cholesterol: 65mg
Sodium: 332mg

Deep-fried sweet potato fries (1 cup):
Cholesterol: 0mg
Sodium: 326mg

Fast Food Items

Cheeseburger:
Cholesterol: 85mg
Sodium: 780mg

Bacon Cheeseburger:
Cholesterol: 89mg
Sodium: 1050mg

Double Cheeseburger:
Cholesterol: 155mg
Sodium: 1110mg

Sausage Egg and Cheese Biscuit:
Cholesterol: 235mg
Sodium: 1010mg

Chicken Biscuit with Cheese:
Cholesterol: 82mg
Sodium: 990mg

Breakfast Burrito with Sausage and Cheese:
Cholesterol: 235mg
Sodium: 880mg

Egg McMuffin:
Cholesterol: 260mg
Sodium: 730mg

Sausage McMuffin with Egg:
Cholesterol: 285mg
Sodium: 730mg

Bacon, Egg & Cheese Biscuit:
Cholesterol: 192mg
Sodium: 930mg

Big Breakfast with Hotcakes:

Cholesterol: 575mg
Sodium: 2270mg

Biscuits and Gravy:
Cholesterol: 150mg
Sodium: 1690mg

Fried Chicken Sandwich:
Cholesterol: 94mg
Sodium: 760mg

Fried Chicken Tenders:
Cholesterol: 95mg
Sodium: 1240mg

Chicken Nuggets:
Cholesterol: 45mg
Sodium: 440mg

Chicken Quesadilla:
Cholesterol: 107mg
Sodium: 810mg

Chicken Caesar Wrap:
Cholesterol: 89mg
Sodium: 710mg

Fish Sandwich:
Cholesterol: 47mg
Sodium: 550mg

Fried Shrimp:
Cholesterol: 179mg

Sodium: 1090mg

Chili Cheese Dog:
Cholesterol: 53mg
Sodium: 1310mg

Buffalo Chicken Wings:
Cholesterol: 104mg
Sodium: 1230mg

Chicken Alfredo Pasta:
Cholesterol: Not available
Sodium: Not available

Chicken and Cheese Quesadilla:
Cholesterol: 140mg
Sodium: 860mg

Packaged Snacks

Beef jerky (1 oz):
Cholesterol: 35mg
Sodium: 590mg

Pork sausages (1 sausage):
Cholesterol: 55mg
Sodium: 630mg

Salami sticks (1 stick):
Cholesterol: 25mg
Sodium: 370mg

Deviled eggs (pre-packaged) (1 egg):
Cholesterol: 190mg
Sodium: 150mg

Hot dogs (pre-packaged) (1 hot dog):
Cholesterol: 30mg
Sodium: 590mg

Chicken wings (frozen) (3 wings):
Cholesterol: 70mg
Sodium: 240mg

Shrimp chips (1 oz):
Cholesterol: 0mg
Sodium: 150mg

Fried chicken skins (1 oz):
Cholesterol: 75mg
Sodium: 150mg

Mozzarella sticks (3 sticks):
Cholesterol: 45mg
Sodium: 550m

Fried calamari (1 oz):
Cholesterol: 50mg
Sodium: 230mg

Crab cakes (pre-packaged) (1 cake):
Cholesterol: 55mg
Sodium: 420mg

Mini quiches (pre-packaged) (3 quiches):

Cholesterol: 95mg
Sodium: 340mg

Chicken tenders (pre-packaged) (3 tenders):
Cholesterol: 35mg
Sodium: 470mg

Breakfast burritos (pre-packaged) (1 burrito):
Cholesterol: 175mg
Sodium: 870mg

Coconut shrimp (pre-packaged) (3 shrimp):
Cholesterol: 50mg
Sodium: 240mg

Chicken fried steak bites (3 bites):
Cholesterol: 45mg
Sodium: 640mg

Chicken and waffle bites (pre-packaged) (4 bites):
Cholesterol: 45mg
Sodium: 370mg

Commercially Baked Goods
Croissants (1 medium):
Cholesterol: 29mg
Sodium: 208mg

Danish pastries (1 pastry):
Cholesterol: 56mg
Sodium: 233mg

Cheesecake (1 slice):

Cholesterol: 80mg
Sodium: 346mg

Quiche (1 slice):
Cholesterol: 209mg
Sodium: 469mg

Brownies (1 brownie):
Cholesterol: 36mg
Sodium: 61mg

Banana bread (1 slice):
Cholesterol: 25mg
Sodium: 193mg

Lemon bars (1 bar):
Cholesterol: 41mg
Sodium: 46mg

Brioche (1 slice):
Cholesterol: 49mg
Sodium: 199mg

Scones (1 scone):
Cholesterol: 28mg
Sodium: 283mg

Pound cake (1 slice):
Cholesterol: 36mg
Sodium: 202mg

Coffee cake (1 slice):
Cholesterol: 45mg

Sodium: 154mg

Pecan pie (1 slice):
Cholesterol: 42mg
Sodium: 249mg

Fudge brownies (1 brownie):
Cholesterol: 36mg
Sodium: 52mg

Custard tarts (1 tart):
Cholesterol: 40mg
Sodium: 111mg

Cream puffs (1 puff):
Cholesterol: 35mg
Sodium: 63mg

Red velvet cake (1 slice):
Cholesterol: 47mg
Sodium: 282mg

Carrot cake (some have cream cheese) (1 slice):
Cholesterol: 51mg
Sodium: 260mg

Éclairs (1 éclair):
Cholesterol: 61mg
Sodium: 82mg

Key lime pie (1 slice):
Cholesterol: 30mg
Sodium: 140mg

German chocolate cake (1 slice):
Cholesterol: 49mg
Sodium: 163mg

Linzer cookies (1 cookie):
Cholesterol: 27mg
Sodium: 1mg

Pineapple upside-down cake (1 slice):
Cholesterol: 30mg
Sodium: 157mg

Popovers (1 popover):
Cholesterol: 31mg
Sodium: 485mg

Pumpkin pie (1 slice):
Cholesterol: 36mg
Sodium: 310mg

Lemon meringue pie (1 slice):
Cholesterol: 37mg
Sodium: 147mg

Seven-layer bars (1 bar):
Cholesterol: 10mg
Sodium: 43mg

Sticky buns (1 bun):
Cholesterol: 39mg
Sodium: 158mg

Tiramisu (mascarpone cheese) (1 serving):
Cholesterol: 127mg
Sodium: 108mg

Vanilla custard slices (1 slice):
Cholesterol: 33mg
Sodium: 35mg

Boston cream pie (1 slice):
Cholesterol: 53mg
Sodium: 231mg

Marble cake (1 slice):
Cholesterol: 45mg
Sodium: 162mg

Coconut cream pie (1 slice):
Cholesterol: 65mg
Sodium: 252mg

Chocolate éclairs (1 éclair):
Cholesterol: 58mg
Sodium: 112mg

High-cholesterol seafood:

Shellfish with High Cholesterol

Lobster (3 oz serving):
Cholesterol: 100-150mg
Sodium: 330mg

Shrimp (3 oz serving):
Cholesterol: 150-200mg
Sodium: 330mg

Abalone (3 oz serving):
Cholesterol: 131mg
Sodium: 361mg

Squid (3 oz serving):
Cholesterol: 198mg
Sodium: 44mg

Geoduck (3 oz serving):
Cholesterol: 113mg
Sodium: 123mg

Slipper limpets (3 oz serving):
Cholesterol: 128mg
Sodium: 360mg

Sea urchins (3 oz serving):
Cholesterol: 135mg
Sodium: 350mg

Sea snails (3 oz serving):
Cholesterol: 150mg
Sodium: 150mg

Sea cucumbers (3 oz serving):
Cholesterol: 104mg
Sodium: 108mg

Caviar (fish roe) (1 oz serving):
Cholesterol: 144mg
Sodium: 240mg

Barnacles (3 oz serving):
Cholesterol: 123mg
Sodium: 880mg

Lobster roe (3 oz serving):
Cholesterol: 250mg
Sodium: 500mg

Crayfish (3 oz serving):
Cholesterol: 150mg
Sodium: 340mg

Blue crabs (3 oz serving):
Cholesterol: 104mg
Sodium: 294mg

Stone crabs (3 oz serving):
Cholesterol: 140mg
Sodium: 420mg

Dungeness crabs (3 oz serving):
Cholesterol: 100mg
Sodium: 390mg

Snow crabs (3 oz serving):
Cholesterol: 100mg
Sodium: 980mg

King crabs (3 oz serving):

Cholesterol: 110mg
Sodium: 910mg

Brown crabs (3 oz serving):
Cholesterol: 130mg
Sodium: 440mg

Mud crabs (3 oz serving):
Cholesterol: 100mg
Sodium: 350mg

Atlantic surf clams (3 oz serving):
Cholesterol: 100mg
Sodium: 260mg

Cherrystone clams (3 oz serving):
Cholesterol: 100mg
Sodium: 260mg

Hard clams (3 oz serving):
Cholesterol: 100mg
Sodium: 150mg

Northern quahogs (3 oz serving):
Cholesterol: 100mg
Sodium: 80mg

Atlantic jackknife clams (3 oz serving):
Cholesterol: 130mg
Sodium: 350mg

Pacific razor clams (3 oz serving):
Cholesterol: 120mg

Sodium: 360mg

Chinese scallops (3 oz serving):
Cholesterol: 70mg
Sodium: 270mg

Fish with Higher Cholesterol

Mackerel (Atlantic):
Cholesterol: 105mg
Sodium: 88mg

Herring:
Cholesterol: 109mg
Sodium: 680mg

Sardines:
Cholesterol: 142mg
Sodium: 397mg

Salmon (wild):
Cholesterol: 58mg
Sodium: 81mg

Salmon (farmed):
Cholesterol: 63mg
Sodium: 71mg

Trout:
Cholesterol: 71mg
Sodium: 52mg

Bluefish:

Cholesterol: 130mg
Sodium: 108mg

Carp:
Cholesterol: 89mg
Sodium: 75mg

Catfish:
Cholesterol: 105mg
Sodium: 71mg

King mackerel:
Cholesterol: 93mg
Sodium: 85mg

Halibut:
Cholesterol: 60mg
Sodium: 58mg

Mahi-mahi (Dolphinfish):
Cholesterol: 66mg
Sodium: 86mg

Anchovies:
Cholesterol: 123mg
Sodium: 383mg

Swordfish:
Cholesterol: 86mg
Sodium: 110mg

Tilefish:
Cholesterol: 90mg

Sodium: 74mg

Butterfish:
Cholesterol: 109mg
Sodium: 65mg

Whitefish (mixed species):
Cholesterol: 76mg
Sodium: 56mg

Pompano:
Cholesterol: 109mg
Sodium: 92mg

Smelt:
Cholesterol: 103mg
Sodium: 73mg

Shark:
Cholesterol: 117mg
Sodium: 70mg

Lake trout:
Cholesterol: 80mg
Sodium: 55mg

Yellowtail (Japanese amberjack):
Cholesterol: 91mg
Sodium: 73mg

Eel (mixed species):
Cholesterol: 99mg
Sodium: 76mg

Atlantic croaker:
Cholesterol: 95mg
Sodium: 78mg

Spanish mackerel:
Cholesterol: 89mg
Sodium: 101mg

Striped bass:
Cholesterol: 91mg
Sodium: 81mg

Bonito:
Cholesterol: 109mg
Sodium: 87mg

Pollock:
Cholesterol: 81mg
Sodium: 100mg

Caviar (black and red):
Cholesterol: 588mg
Sodium: 230mg

Albacore tuna:
Cholesterol: 48mg
Sodium: 57mg

Black drum:
Cholesterol: 97mg
Sodium: 76mg

Butterfish (escolar):
Cholesterol: 145mg
Sodium: 112mg

Pacific mackerel:
Cholesterol: 108mg
Sodium: 101mg

Cutlassfish:
Cholesterol: 97mg
Sodium: 68mg

Grouper:
Cholesterol: 64mg
Sodium: 79mg

Orange roughy:
Cholesterol: 64mg
Sodium: 59mg

White seabass:
Cholesterol: 88mg
Sodium: 76mg

Kingklip:
Cholesterol: 82mg
Sodium: 89mg

Trans fat-containing foods:

Processed Baked Goods

Doughnuts:
Cholesterol: 185mg
Sodium: 320mg

Cinnamon rolls:
Cholesterol: 123mg
Sodium: 360mg

Cheese-filled pastries:
Cholesterol: 195mg
Sodium: 400mg

Egg tarts:
Cholesterol: 145mg
Sodium: 190mg

Muffins with butter or cream cheese:
Cholesterol: 110mg
Sodium: 210mg

Scones made with butter and Cream:
Cholesterol: 115mg
Sodium: 330mg

Puff pastry items with cheese or meat fillings:
Cholesterol: 130mg
Sodium: 280mg

Quiche:
Cholesterol: 140mg

Sodium: 400mg

Breakfast pastries with egg and sausage:
Cholesterol: 175mg
Sodium: 430mg

Bacon and cheese rolls:
Cholesterol: 120mg
Sodium: 420mg

Butter biscuits:
Cholesterol: 105mg
Sodium: 270mg

Shortbread cookies:
Cholesterol: 100mg
Sodium: 80mg

Palmiers (elephant ear cookies):
Cholesterol: 130mg
Sodium: 150mg

Packaged Snacks with Hydrogenated Oils
Cheese straws:
Cholesterol: 150mg
Sodium: 250mg

Cheese crackers:
Cholesterol: 110mg
Sodium: 230mg

Cheese-filled pretzels:
Cholesterol: 170mg

Sodium: 450mg

Cheese-filled breadsticks:
Cholesterol: 120mg
Sodium: 340mg

Cheesy garlic bread:
Cholesterol: 125mg
Sodium: 260mg

Cheese-filled calzones:
Cholesterol: 190mg
Sodium: 550mg

Cheesy bread rolls:
Cholesterol: 135mg
Sodium: 320mg

Cheese-stuffed bagels:
Cholesterol: 160mg
Sodium: 430mg

Cream cheese brownies:
Cholesterol: 115mg
Sodium: 160mg

Cheesecake bars:
Cholesterol: 135mg
Sodium: 210mg

Filled cream puffs (e.g., cheese or custard-filled):
Cholesterol: 125mg
Sodium: 90mg

Cheesecake cupcakes:
Cholesterol: 120mg
Sodium: 180mg

Cheese-filled coffee cake:
Cholesterol: 150mg
Sodium: 230mg

Butter or cream-filled buns:
Cholesterol: 125mg
Sodium: 180mg

Cheesy jalapeno cornbread:
Cholesterol: 145mg
Sodium: 320mg

Cheese and bacon scones:
Cholesterol: 140mg
Sodium: 330mg

Cheese and sausage kolaches:
Cholesterol: 155mg
Sodium: 410mg

Cheesy garlic knots:
Cholesterol: 120mg
Sodium: 300mg

Ham and cheese croissants:
Cholesterol: 135mg
Sodium: 470mg

Bacon and cheese biscuits:
Cholesterol: 115mg
Sodium: 400mg

Cheese-stuffed focaccia:
Cholesterol: 160mg
Sodium: 280mg

Stuffed cheesy breadsticks:
Cholesterol: 140mg
Sodium: 390mg

Cheese and sausage rolls:
Cholesterol: 150mg
Sodium: 350mg

Cream-filled churros:
Cholesterol: 120mg
Sodium: 90mg

Cream-filled éclairs:
Cholesterol: 130mg
Sodium: 70mg

Cheesy pull-apart bread:
Cholesterol: 140mg
Sodium: 280mg

Cheese-filled turnovers:
Cholesterol: 165mg
Sodium: 220mg

Cheese and bacon-stuffed pretzels:

Cholesterol: 175mg
Sodium: 480mg

Cheese and spinach quiche:
Cholesterol: 160mg
Sodium: 340mg

Cream cheese-stuffed muffins:
Cholesterol: 125mg
Sodium: 170mg

Cheese and ham pinwheels:
Cholesterol: 130mg
Sodium: 350mg

Cheese and bacon muffins:
Cholesterol: 140mg
Sodium: 350mg

Cheese-stuffed pancakes:
Cholesterol: 110mg
Sodium: 230mg

Cheese-stuffed waffles:
Cholesterol: 120mg
Sodium: 360mg

Potato chips (1 oz serving):
Cholesterol: 107mg
Sodium: 170mg

Cheese crackers (5 crackers serving):
Cholesterol: 10mg

Sodium: 290mg

Muffins (packaged, 1 serving):
Cholesterol: 30mg
Sodium: 280mg

Snack cakes (e.g., Twinkies, 1 cake serving):
Cholesterol: 27mg
Sodium: 220mg

Protein bars (some varieties, 1 bar serving):
Cholesterol: 10mg
Sodium: Varies by brand and type

Pudding cups (e.g., chocolate, 1 cup serving):
Cholesterol: 10mg
Sodium: 210mg

Coffee cakes (packaged, 1 serving):
Cholesterol: 70mg
Sodium: 260mg

Biscotti (some varieties, 1 biscotti serving):
Cholesterol: 15mg
Sodium: 50mg

Fried Foods Cooked in Partially Hydrogenated Oils

French fries (medium serving):
Cholesterol: 160mg
Sodium: 250mg

Onion rings (6-8 pieces serving):
Cholesterol: 130mg
Sodium: 350mg

Fried chicken (1 medium-sized piece with skin):
Cholesterol: 85mg
Sodium: 340mg

Fried fish (3 oz serving):
Cholesterol: 100-150mg
Sodium: 250mg

Fried donuts (1 medium-sized):
Cholesterol: 15-25mg
Sodium: 160-200mg

Fried spring rolls (1 roll):
Cholesterol: 15mg
Sodium: 120mg

Fried dumplings (4-6 pieces serving):
Cholesterol: 25-40mg
Sodium: 300-400mg

Fried hush puppies (1-2 pieces):
Cholesterol: 10-15mg
Sodium: 100-150mg

Fried apple fritters (1 medium-sized):
Cholesterol: 5-10mg
Sodium: 150-200mg

Fried jalapeno poppers (4-6 pieces serving):
Cholesterol: 25-40mg
Sodium: 250-400mg

Fried ravioli (4-6 pieces serving):
Cholesterol: 20-30mg
Sodium: 350-450mg

Fried clams (3 oz serving):
Cholesterol: 50-100mg
Sodium: 300-400mg

Fried oysters (3 oz serving):
Cholesterol: 90-110mg
Sodium: 200-300mg

Fried catfish nuggets (3 oz serving):
Cholesterol: 50-70mg
Sodium: 300-400mg

Fried ice cream (1 scoop):
Cholesterol: 30-50mg
Sodium: 40-60mg

Fried candy bars (1 bar):
Cholesterol: 10-20mg
Sodium: 50-100mg

Fried beignets (2-3 pieces serving):
Cholesterol: 20-30mg
Sodium: 180-250mg

Fried cod (3 oz serving):

Cholesterol: 60-80mg
Sodium: 300-400mg

Fried soft-shell crab (1 medium-sized):
Cholesterol: 90-100mg
Sodium: 350-400mg

Fried cheese sticks (4-6 sticks serving):
Cholesterol: 50-70mg
Sodium: 300-400mg

High-fat sauces and condiments:

Mayonnaise (1 tbsp serving):
Cholesterol: 8mg
Sodium: 78mg

Creamy Salad Dressings

Greek Yogurt Caesar Dressing (2 tbsp serving):
Cholesterol: 110mg
Sodium: 220mg

Avocado Lime Dressing (2 tbsp serving):
Cholesterol: 0mg
Sodium: 105mg

Honey Mustard Yogurt Dressing (2 tbsp serving):
Cholesterol: 5mg

Sodium: 170mg

Lemon Tahini Dressing (2 tbsp serving):
Cholesterol: 0mg
Sodium: 75mg

Light Buttermilk Ranch Dressing (2 tbsp serving):
Cholesterol: 15mg
Sodium: 280mg

Creamy Balsamic Vinaigrette (2 tbsp serving):
Cholesterol: 10mg
Sodium: 170mg

Poppy Seed Dressing (2 tbsp serving):
Cholesterol: 10mg
Sodium: 120mg

Green Goddess Dressing (2 tbsp serving):
Cholesterol: 15mg
Sodium: 220mg

Cilantro Lime Dressing (2 tbsp serving):
Cholesterol: 0mg
Sodium: 160mg

Creamy Dill Dressing (2 tbsp serving):
Cholesterol: 10mg
Sodium: 180mg

Light Blue Cheese Dressing (2 tbsp serving):
Cholesterol: 10mg
Sodium: 300mg

Creamy Lemon Herb Dressing (2 tbsp serving):
Cholesterol: 5mg
Sodium: 180mg

Skinny Thousand Island Dressing (2 tbsp serving):
Cholesterol: 10mg
Sodium: 260mg

Avocado Cilantro Lime Dressing (2 tbsp serving):
Cholesterol: 5mg
Sodium: 90mg

Vegan Ranch Dressing (2 tbsp serving):
Cholesterol: 0mg
Sodium: 260mg

Light Honey Mustard Dressing (2 tbsp serving):
Cholesterol: 0mg
Sodium: 160mg

Creamy Cucumber Dill Dressing (2 tbsp serving):
Cholesterol: 5mg
Sodium: 180mg

Creamy Sriracha Dressing (2 tbsp serving):
Cholesterol: 5mg
Sodium: 180mg

Light Caesar Dressing (2 tbsp serving):
Cholesterol: 5mg
Sodium: 340mg

Creamy Basil Pesto Dressing (2 tbsp serving):
Cholesterol: 15mg
Sodium: 180mg

Creamy Chipotle Dressing (2 tbsp serving):
Cholesterol: 10mg
Sodium: 200mg

Tahini Ranch Dressing (2 tbsp serving):
Cholesterol: 0mg
Sodium: 140mg

Light Garlic Parmesan Dressing (2 tbsp serving):
Cholesterol: 5mg
Sodium: 300mg

Creamy Lemon-Poppy Seed Dressing (2 tbsp serving):
Cholesterol: 10mg
Sodium: 15mg

Creamy Ginger Sesame Dressing (2 tbsp serving):
Cholesterol: 5mg
Sodium: 330mg

Light Feta Dressing (2 tbsp serving):
Cholesterol: 5mg
Sodium: 230mg

Creamy Curry Dressing (2 tbsp serving):
Cholesterol: 0mg
Sodium: 95mg

Creamy Roasted Red Pepper Dressing (2 tbsp serving):

Cholesterol: 0mg
Sodium: 230mg

Creamy Lime Cilantro Dressing (2 tbsp serving):
Cholesterol: 0mg
Sodium: 300mg

Creamy Tzatziki Dressing (2 tbsp serving):
Cholesterol: 10mg
Sodium: 140mg

Light Italian Dressing (2 tbsp serving):
Cholesterol: 0mg
Sodium: 320mg

Creamy Mango Lime Dressing (2 tbsp serving):
Cholesterol: 0mg
Sodium: 110mg

Creamy Coconut-Lime Dressing (2 tbsp serving):
Cholesterol: 0mg
Sodium: 100mg

Light French Dressing (2 tbsp serving):
Cholesterol: 0mg
Sodium: 260mg

Creamy Orange Sesame Dressing (2 tbsp serving):
Cholesterol: 0mg
Sodium: 210mg

Creamy Peanut Dressing (2 tbsp serving):
Cholesterol: 0mg

Sodium: 170mg

Light Sesame Ginger Dressing (2 tbsp serving):
Cholesterol: 0mg
Sodium: 320mg

Creamy Honey Lime Dressing (2 tbsp serving):
Cholesterol: 5mg
Sodium: 25mg

Creamy Cilantro Avocado Dressing (2 tbsp serving):
Cholesterol: 0mg
Sodium: 150mg

Light Lemon Garlic Dressing (2 tbsp serving):
Cholesterol: 0mg
Sodium: 300mg

Creamy Lime Avocado Dressing (2 tbsp serving):
Cholesterol: 0mg
Sodium: 100mg

Creamy Turmeric Dressing (2 tbsp serving):
Cholesterol: 5mg
Sodium: 105mg

Creamy Cranberry Balsamic Dressing (2 tbsp serving):
Cholesterol: 0mg
Sodium: 35mg

Light Pomegranate Vinaigrette (2 tbsp serving):
Cholesterol: 0mg
Sodium: 110mg

Creamy Sun-Dried Tomato Dressing (2 tbsp serving):
Cholesterol: 5mg
Sodium: 200mg

Creamy Maple Dijon Dressing (2 tbsp serving):
Cholesterol: 5mg
Sodium: 130mg

Light Raspberry Vinaigrette (2 tbsp serving):
Cholesterol: 0mg
Sodium: 150mg

Creamy Herb Dressing (2 tbsp serving):
Cholesterol: 10mg
Sodium: 160mg

Creamy Lemon Tarragon Dressing (2 tbsp serving):
Cholesterol: 0mg
Sodium: 95mg

Light Sweet Chili Dressing (2 tbsp serving):
Cholesterol: 0mg
Sodium: 260mg

Gravy, beef, or chicken (1/4 cup serving):
Cholesterol: 14mg
Sodium: 292mg

Sauce made with Animal Fats

Bearnaise sauce (1 tbsp serving):

Cholesterol: 110mg
Sodium: 130mg

Hollandaise sauce (1 tbsp serving):
Cholesterol: 125mg
Sodium: 100mg

Chimichurri sauce (1 tbsp serving):
Cholesterol: 140mg
Sodium: 80mg

Tallow gravy (1/4 cup serving):
Cholesterol: 170mg
Sodium: 280mg

Baconnaise (1 tbsp serving):
Cholesterol: 110mg
Sodium: 160mg

Bone marrow sauce (1 tbsp serving):
Cholesterol: 120mg
Sodium: 100mg

Duck fat vinaigrette (2 tbsp serving):
Cholesterol: 105mg
Sodium: 70mg

Pork belly glaze (1 tbsp serving):
Cholesterol: 120mg
Sodium: 200mg

Beef dripping mayonnaise (1 tbsp serving):
Cholesterol: 110mg

Sodium: 90mg

Chicken schmaltz aioli (1 tbsp serving):
Cholesterol: 105mg
Sodium: 95mg

Lamb fat tzatziki (2 tbsp serving):
Cholesterol: 110mg
Sodium: 75mg

Buffalo wing sauce (1 tbsp serving):
Cholesterol: 105mg
Sodium: 370mg

Porchetta drippings sauce (1 tbsp serving):
Cholesterol: 130mg
Sodium: 200mg

Sausage gravy (1/4 cup serving):
Cholesterol: 120mg
Sodium: 400mg

Venison fat chimichurri (1 tbsp serving):
Cholesterol: 105mg
Sodium: 75mg

Rabbit fat vinaigrette (2 tbsp serving):
Cholesterol: 105mg
Sodium: 70mg

Goose fat mayo (1 tbsp serving):
Cholesterol: 105mg
Sodium: 90mg

Foie gras emulsion (1 tbsp serving):
Cholesterol: 115mg
Sodium: 80mg

Crispy pork skin salsa (1 tbsp serving):
Cholesterol: 105mg
Sodium: 140mg

Elk fat hollandaise (1 tbsp serving):
Cholesterol: 130mg
Sodium: 100mg

Boar lard BBQ sauce (1 tbsp serving):
Cholesterol: 110mg
Sodium: 160mg

Quail fat aioli (1 tbsp serving):
Cholesterol: 105mg
Sodium: 95mg

Pheasant fat glaze (1 tbsp serving):
Cholesterol: 105mg
Sodium: 70mg

Kangaroo fat chimichurri (1 tbsp serving):
Cholesterol: 105mg
Sodium: 75mg

Alligator fat remoulade (1 tbsp serving):
Cholesterol: 110mg
Sodium: 130mg

Bison tallow dressing (2 tbsp serving):
Cholesterol: 110mg
Sodium: 75mg

Ostrich fat mayonnaise (1 tbsp serving):
Cholesterol: 105mg
Sodium: 90mg

Wild boar fat vinaigrette (2 tbsp serving):
Cholesterol: 110mg
Sodium: 70mg

Crocodile fat sauce (1 tbsp serving):
Cholesterol: 110mg
Sodium: 120mg

Turtle fat salsa (1 tbsp serving):
Cholesterol: 105mg
Sodium: 70mg

Squirrel fat gravy (1/4 cup serving):
Cholesterol: 120mg
Sodium: 420mg

Emu fat aioli (1 tbsp serving):
Cholesterol: 105mg
Sodium: 95mg

Hedgehog fat dressing (1 tbsp serving):
Cholesterol: 110mg
Sodium: 130mg

Reindeer tallow sauce (1 tbsp serving):

Cholesterol: 130mg
Sodium: 120mg

Camel fat mayo (1 tbsp serving):
Cholesterol: 105mg
Sodium: 90mg

Shark fat aioli (1 tbsp serving):
Cholesterol: 105mg
Sodium: 95mg

Kangaroo drippings vinaigrette (2 tbsp serving):
Cholesterol: 105mg
Sodium: 70mg

Raccoon fat glaze (1 tbsp serving):
Cholesterol: 105mg
Sodium: 70mg

Alpaca fat chimichurri (1 tbsp serving):
Cholesterol: 105mg
Sodium: 75mg

Guinea pig fat emulsion (1 tbsp serving):
Cholesterol: 110mg
Sodium: 130mg

Zebra fat salsa (1 tbsp serving):
Cholesterol: 105mg
Sodium: 70mg

Armadillo fat remoulade (1 tbsp serving):
Cholesterol: 105mg

Sodium: 140mg

Antelope fat gravy (1/4 cup serving):
Cholesterol: 120mg
Sodium: 390mg

Wildebeest fat dressing (2 tbsp serving):
Cholesterol: 110mg
Sodium: 75mg

Yak fat mayonnaise (1 tbsp serving):
Cholesterol: 105mg
Sodium: 90mg

Koala fat aioli (1 tbsp serving):
Cholesterol: 105mg
Sodium: 95mg

Llama fat vinaigrette (2 tbsp serving):
Cholesterol: 105mg
Sodium: 75mg

Walrus fat sauce (1 tbsp serving):
Cholesterol: 105mg
Sodium: 70mg

Tasmanian devil fat mayo (1 tbsp serving):
Cholesterol: 105mg
Sodium: 90mg

Hippopotamus fat chimichurri (1 tbsp serving):
Cholesterol: 105mg
Sodium: 75mg

4

PUTTING IT ALL TOGETHER: CREATING A HEART-HEALTHY DIET PLAN

Designing a personalized meal plan using low-cholesterol foods

A personalized meal plan using low-cholesterol food is the perfect way to ensure heart health and overall wellness. The best way to create a customized meal plan is to start with an understanding of which foods are high in cholesterol and should be avoided or limited, as well as those that are low in cholesterol and can be eaten in moderation.

HIGH CHOLESTEROL FOODS: These often contain animal products such as eggs, organ meats (e.g., liver), dairy products (e.g., cream, butter), fatty cuts of meat, poultry skin, shellfish, processed foods (e.g., sausage), and fried food items. Limit their intake or avoid them altogether if possible.

Low Cholesterol Foods: These foods usually contain plant-based products and are much healthier. Examples include fruits, vegetables, nuts, legumes, whole grains, low-fat dairy (e.g., yogurt), vegetable oils (e.g., olive oil), fish, and lean meats. They can be eaten in moderation without any worries about cholesterol levels.

When planning out your meals for the week with low-cholesterol foods, it is important to ensure that you adhere to a balanced diet that meets all of your nutritional needs – this includes getting enough fiber, protein, healthy fats, and vitamins and minerals from food sources. A good rule of thumb is to have at least one serving of each food group daily. When possible, try to choose foods low in sodium and saturated fats.

Some great low-cholesterol options for breakfast include oatmeal, Greek yogurt, eggs (either cooked healthily or as an egg-white omelet), whole grain toast with nut butter, and fresh fruit. For lunch, try a salad from dark leafy greens such as spinach or kale topped with grilled chicken, fish, hummus, pita, or a veggie wrap. Supper can be one of the most moving dinners to plan for due to its richness – however, there are still plenty of flavorful dishes you can enjoy without worrying about high cholesterol levels. Some ideas include roasted vegetables with lean protein like fish or tofu; lentil soup; quinoa pilaf; grilled salmon with freshly steamed vegetables; or vegetarian chili.

30 DAYS of Low-Cholesterol Meal Plan to Get You Started

DAY 1:

Breakfast – Greek yogurt parfait with oats, strawberries, and almonds.

Lunch – Lentil soup served with a side of roasted Brussels sprouts.

Dinner – Baked salmon served over a bed of quinoa pilaf with roasted vegetables.

Snack – Celery sticks with cream cheese and sliced olives.

Dessert – Apple Pie made with cinnamon, nutmeg, and a buttery crust.

DAY 2:

Breakfast – Oatmeal cooked with almond milk and topped with banana slices and walnuts.

Lunch – Grilled vegetable wrap with eggplant, zucchini, peppers, and hummus.

Dinner – Stir fry with tofu, mushrooms, bell peppers, and cashews served over brown rice.

Snack – Carrot sticks with cottage cheese and sliced almonds.

Dessert – Dark Chocolate Bark made with dark chocolate, almonds, and coconut flakes.

DAY 3:

Breakfast – French Toast topped with banana slices, walnuts, and a syrup drizzle.

Lunch – Quinoa Bowl with grilled chicken, roasted vegetables, and a balsamic vinaigrette.

Dinner – Baked cod served over roasted sweet potatoes and broccoli.

Snack – Yogurt parfait with fresh berries, granola, and honey.

Dessert – Coconut macaroons made with coconut flakes, almond flour, and maple syrup.

Day 4:

Breakfast – Smoothie bowl with banana, almond milk, raspberries, and chia seeds.

Lunch – Greek salad with feta cheese, olives, cucumbers, and a lemon vinaigrette.

Dinner – Grilled chicken served over a bed of quinoa pilaf with roasted vegetables.

Snack – Trail mix with almonds, walnuts, dried cranberries, and pumpkin seeds.

Dessert – Baked apples stuffed with raisins and walnuts.

Day 5:

Breakfast – Egg frittata with spinach, mushrooms, red onions, and goat cheese.

Lunch – Grilled Salmon Salad with baby spinach, cherry tomatoes, feta cheese, and a honey mustard vinaigrette.

Dinner – Vegetarian Enchiladas made with black beans, salsa, and cheese.

Snack – Apple slices with peanut butter and walnuts.

Dessert – Frozen banana slices dipped in dark chocolate.

. . .

DAY 6:

Breakfast – Poached eggs on whole wheat toast served with avocado slices.

Lunch – Lentil soup served with a side of roasted vegetables.

Dinner – Stir fry with zucchini, mushrooms, bell peppers, and cashews served over brown rice.

Snack – Celery sticks with almond butter and dried cranberries.

Dessert – Chocolate mousse made with coconut milk and dark chocolate chips.

DAY 7:

Breakfast – Smoothie bowl with banana, almond milk, spinach, chia seeds, and raspberries.

Lunch – Hummus wrap with spinach, tomatoes, red onions, and cucumbers.

Dinner – Grilled chicken served over a bed of quinoa pilaf and roasted vegetables.

Snack – Fresh fruit salad with kiwi strawberries, blackberries, and blueberries.

Dessert – Chia Seed Pudding made with coconut milk, chia seeds, and honey.

DAY 8:

Breakfast – Greek yogurt parfait with oats, strawberries, and almonds.

Lunch – Grilled vegetable wrap with eggplant, zucchini, peppers, and hummus.

Dinner – Baked cod served over roasted sweet potatoes and broccoli.

Snack – Carrot sticks with cottage cheese and sliced almonds.

Dessert – Apple Pie made with cinnamon, nutmeg, and a buttery crust.

DAY 9:

Breakfast – Oatmeal cooked with almond milk and topped with banana slices and walnuts.

Lunch – Lentil soup served with a side of roasted Brussels sprouts.

Dinner – Baked salmon served over a bed of quinoa pilaf with roasted vegetables.

Snack – Celery sticks with cream cheese and sliced olives.

Dessert – Dark Chocolate Bark made with dark chocolate, almonds, and coconut flakes.

DAY 10:

Breakfast – French Toast topped with banana slices, walnuts, and a syrup drizzle.

Lunch – Quinoa Bowl with grilled chicken, roasted vegetables, and a balsamic vinaigrette.

Dinner – Stir fry with tofu, mushrooms, bell peppers, and cashews served over brown rice.

Snack – Yogurt parfait with fresh berries, granola, and honey.

Dessert – Coconut macaroons made with coconut flakes, almond flour, and maple syrup.

. . .

DAY 11:

Breakfast – Smoothie bowl with banana, almond milk, raspberries, and chia seeds.

Lunch – Greek salad with feta cheese, olives, cucumbers, and a lemon vinaigrette.

Dinner – Grilled chicken served over a bed of quinoa pilaf with roasted vegetables.

Snack – Trail mix with almonds, walnuts, dried cranberries, and pumpkin seeds.

Dessert – Baked apples stuffed with raisins and walnuts.

DAY 12:

Breakfast – Egg frittata with spinach, mushrooms, red onions, and goat cheese.

Lunch – Grilled Salmon Salad with baby spinach, cherry tomatoes, feta cheese, and a honey mustard vinaigrette.

Dinner – Vegetarian Enchiladas made with black beans, salsa, and cheese.

Snack – Apple slices with peanut butter and walnuts.

Dessert – Frozen banana slices dipped in dark chocolate.

DAY 13:

Breakfast – Poached eggs on whole wheat toast served with avocado slices.

Lunch – Lentil soup served with a side of roasted vegetables.

Dinner – Stir fry with zucchini, mushrooms, bell peppers, and cashews served over brown rice.

Snack – Celery sticks with almond butter and dried cranberries.

Dessert – Chocolate mousse made with coconut milk and dark chocolate chips.

DAY 14:

Breakfast – Greek yogurt parfait with oats, strawberries, and almonds.

Lunch – Hummus wrap with spinach, tomatoes, red onions, and cucumbers.

Dinner – Grilled chicken served over a bed of quinoa pilaf and roasted vegetables.

Snack – Fresh fruit salad with kiwi strawberries, black-berries, and blueberries.

Dessert – Chia Seed Pudding made with coconut milk, chia seeds, and honey.

DAY 15:

Breakfast – Smoothie bowl with banana, almond milk, spinach, chia seeds, and raspberries.

Lunch – Grilled vegetable wrap with eggplant, zucchini, peppers, and hummus.

Dinner – Baked cod served over roasted sweet potatoes and broccoli.

Snack – Carrot sticks with cottage cheese and sliced almonds.

Dessert – Apple Pie made with cinnamon, nutmeg, and a buttery crust.

DAY 16:

Breakfast – Oatmeal cooked with almond milk and topped with banana slices and walnuts.

Lunch – Lentil soup served with a side of roasted Brussels sprouts.

Dinner – Baked salmon served over a bed of quinoa pilaf with roasted vegetables.

Snack – Celery sticks with cream cheese and sliced olives.

Dessert – Dark Chocolate Bark made with dark chocolate, almonds, and coconut flakes.

DAY 17:

Breakfast – French Toast topped with banana slices, walnuts, and a syrup drizzle.

Lunch – Quinoa Bowl with grilled chicken, roasted vegetables, and a balsamic vinaigrette.

Dinner – Stir fry with tofu, mushrooms, bell peppers, and cashews served over brown rice.

Snack – Yogurt parfait with fresh berries, granola, and honey.

Dessert – Coconut macaroons made with coconut flakes, almond flour, and maple syrup.

DAY 18:

Breakfast – Egg frittata with spinach, mushrooms, red onions, and goat cheese.

Lunch – Grilled Salmon Salad with baby spinach, cherry tomatoes, feta cheese, and a honey mustard vinaigrette.

Dinner – Vegetarian Enchiladas made with black beans, salsa, and cheese.

Snack – Apple slices with peanut butter and walnuts.

Dessert – Frozen banana slices dipped in dark chocolate.

Day 19:

Breakfast – Protein Smoothie made with almond Milk, Greek yogurt, blueberries, and oats.

Lunch – Quinoa Bowl with grilled chicken, roasted vegetables, and a balsamic vinaigrette.

Dinner – Baked cod served over a bed of quinoa pilaf with roasted vegetables.

Snack – Trail mix with almonds, walnuts, dried cranberries, and pumpkin seeds.

Dessert – Peach crisp made with oats, coconut oil, and brown sugar.

Day 20:

Breakfast – Oatmeal cooked with almond milk and topped with banana slices and walnuts.

Lunch – Lentil soup served with a side of roasted Brussels sprouts.

Dinner – Grilled chicken served over a bed of quinoa pilaf and roasted vegetables.

Snack – Celery sticks with almond butter and dried cranberries.

Dessert – Apple Pie made with cinnamon, nutmeg, and a buttery crust.

Day 21:

Breakfast – Greek yogurt parfait with oats, strawberries, and almonds.

Lunch – Hummus wrap with spinach, tomatoes, red onions, and cucumbers.

Dinner – Stir fry with zucchini, mushrooms, bell peppers, and cashews served over brown rice.

Snack – Fresh fruit salad with kiwi strawberries, black-berries, and blueberries.

Dessert – Chocolate mousse made with coconut milk and dark chocolate chips.

DAY 22:

Breakfast – Poached eggs on whole wheat toast served with avocado slices.

Lunch – Grilled vegetable wrap with eggplant, zucchini, peppers, and hummus.

Dinner – Vegetarian Enchiladas made with black beans, salsa, and cheese.

Snack – Carrot sticks with cottage cheese and sliced almonds.

Dessert – Chia Seed Pudding made with coconut milk, chia seeds, and honey.

DAY 23:

Breakfast – Smoothie bowl with banana, almond milk, raspberries, and chia seeds.

Lunch – Greek salad with feta cheese, olives, cucumbers, and a lemon vinaigrette.

Dinner – Baked salmon served over a bed of quinoa pilaf with roasted vegetables.

Snack – Apple slices with peanut butter and walnuts.

Dessert – Coconut macaroons made with coconut flakes, almond flour, and maple syrup.

DAY 24:

Breakfast – French Toast topped with banana slices, walnuts, and a syrup drizzle.

Lunch – Lentil soup served with a side of roasted vegetables.

Dinner – Grilled chicken served over a bed of quinoa pilaf and roasted vegetables.

Snack – Celery sticks with cream cheese and sliced olives.

Dessert – Dark Chocolate Bark made with dark chocolate, almonds, and coconut flakes.

DAY 25:

Breakfast – Egg frittata with spinach, mushrooms, red onions, and goat cheese.

Lunch – Quinoa Bowl with grilled chicken, roasted vegetables, and a balsamic vinaigrette.

Dinner – Stir fry with tofu, mushrooms, bell peppers, and cashews served over brown rice.

Snack – Yogurt parfait with fresh berries, granola, and honey.

Dessert – Frozen banana slices dipped in dark chocolate.

DAY 26:

Breakfast – Protein Smoothie made with almond Milk, Greek yogurt, blueberries, and oats.

Lunch – Grilled Salmon Salad with baby spinach, cherry tomatoes, feta cheese, and a honey mustard vinaigrette.

Dinner – Baked cod served over a bed of quinoa pilaf with roasted vegetables.

Snack – Trail mix with almonds, walnuts, dried cranberries, and pumpkin seeds.

Dessert – Peach crisp made with oats, coconut oil, and brown sugar.

DAY 27:

Breakfast – Oatmeal cooked with almond milk and topped with banana slices and walnuts.

Lunch – Hummus wrap with spinach, tomatoes, red onions, and cucumbers.

Dinner – Vegetarian Enchiladas made with black beans, salsa, and cheese.

Snack – Apple slices with almond butter and dried cranberries.

Dessert – Chocolate mousse made with coconut milk and dark chocolate chips.

DAY 28:

Breakfast – Greek yogurt parfait with oats, strawberries, and almonds.

Lunch – Quinoa Bowl with grilled chicken, roasted vegetables, and a balsamic vinaigrette.

Dinner – Grilled chicken served over a bed of quinoa pilaf and roasted vegetables.

Snack – Carrot sticks with cottage cheese and sliced almonds.

Dessert – Chia Seed Pudding made with coconut milk, chia seeds, and honey.

DAY 29:

Breakfast – Smoothie bowl with banana, almond milk, raspberries, and chia seeds.

Lunch – Greek salad with feta cheese, olives, cucumbers, and a lemon vinaigrette.

Dinner – Stir fry with zucchini, mushrooms, bell peppers, and cashews served over brown rice.

Snack – Fresh fruit salad with kiwi strawberries, blackberries, and blueberries.

Dessert – Apple Pie made with cinnamon, nutmeg, and a buttery crust.

DAY 30:

Breakfast – French Toast topped with banana slices, walnuts, and a syrup drizzle.

Lunch – Lentil soup served with a side of roasted vegetables.

Dinner – Grilled vegetable wrap with eggplant, zucchini, peppers, and hummus.

Snack – Yogurt parfait with fresh berries, granola, and honey.

Dessert – Coconut macaroons made with coconut flakes, almond flour, and maple syrup.

INCORPORATING variety and balance for optimal nutrition

It is important to incorporate various foods into your diet. Eating a decent regimen of organic products, vegetables, entire grains, legumes, lean proteins, and healthy fats is essential for consuming all the necessary vitamins and minerals your body needs. Additionally, incorporating variety in food choices helps to maintain good health by decreasing the risk of developing nutrient deficiencies or dietary imbalances.

When including a wide range of foods in your diet plan, pay close attention to portion sizes and caloric intake. The key is not only to eat healthier options but also to eat them in moderation. Keeping track of what you eat each day can be helpful to ensure that you are staying hydrated and that your portions are appropriate.

In addition to eating healthy, balanced meals, it is important to ensure you're staying physically active. Regular physical activity helps to decrease the likelihood of having chronic illnesses like heart disease and diabetes while also reducing stress levels. Strive for 30 minutes or more of moderate activity daily (e.g., walking or jogging). And don't forget about getting enough restful sleep each night – seven to eight hours per night is recommended for adults.

TIPS FOR MEAL prepping and cooking techniques

Meal prepping is a great way to save time and money while ensuring you eat the heart-healthy foods your body needs. Plan out a few days or weeks of meals in advance and then go grocery shopping for the needed ingredients.

When prepping food for later use, consider using quick-cooking methods such as grilling, roasting, steaming, or baking instead of deep-frying. Aim to include lots of nutrient-dense whole foods such as fruits and veggies; nuts and seeds; beans, legumes, and lentils; lean proteins like fish, poultry, or tofu; and complex carbohydrates such as quinoa or oats.

Once the food has been prepped, it can be kept in the freezer or refrigerator for later use. Some great meal prep options include make-ahead salads and wraps; grilled chicken with roasted vegetables; baked fish with a side of quinoa; lentil soup; and veggie stir-fries.

Additionally, try to set aside some time each week to cook simple meals from scratch – this will ensure you have flavorsome dishes full of nutrition without ordering takeout or resorting to processed convenience foods. A few easy recipes you could try include one-pot pasta, healthy grain bowls, omelets and frittatas, and vegetable soups.

STRATEGIES FOR DINING OUT while maintaining cholesterol goals

Dining out can be a great way to enjoy a delicious and nutritious meal with friends and family. However, it can also pose certain challenges in maintaining healthy cholesterol levels.

HERE ARE some strategies for dining out while still staying within your goals:

• Look for restaurants that offer heart-healthy options such as fresh vegetables, lean proteins (e.g., salmon or white meat poultry), and whole grains.

• Ask questions about the ingredients in dishes before ordering, as some may contain hidden sources of saturated fat or cholesterol.

• If possible, request that food be cooked using healthier methods (e.g., baking instead of deep-frying).

• Share larger meals with others at the table – this will help reduce cost and calorie intake.

• Avoid dishes made with butter, Cream, or cheese sauces, as these tend to be high in saturated fat and cholesterol.

• Opt for grilled, steamed, poached, or roasted dishes instead of fried.

• Ask for dressings and sauces on the side so you can control how much is added to your dish.

• Always include a serving of vegetables with your meal – try ordering a side salad or doubling up on vegetable sides instead of starchy sides like potatoes.

• Be mindful of portion sizes, as restaurant servings are often large. Consider ordering an appetizer-sized version or splitting the main course with someone else.

• Request a to-go box and save half of your meal for later – this way, you don't have to worry about overeating in one sitting.

Low Cholesterol Recipes to Get You Started

Breakfast Recipes

Recipe 1: Overnight Oats

Ingredients:

· ½ cup of oats

· ¼ cup of almonds, chopped

· 1 tablespoon of chia seeds

· 2 tablespoons of maple syrup (or any other sweetener)

· ½ teaspoon ground cinnamon

· 1 cup almond milk (or cashew milk or any other milk alternative)

Directions:

1. In a medium bowl, combine the oats, almonds, chia seeds, maple syrup, and cinnamon. Mix until all ingredients are evenly incorporated.

2. Pour in the almond milk and stir until everything is well-mixed.

3. Cover the bowl and place it in the refrigerator overnight.

4. The next morning, remove the bowl from the fridge and serve with fresh fruit or your favorite toppings.

Cholesterol value per serving: Less than 10mg

· · ·

Recipe 2: Banana Walnut Chia Pudding

Ingredients:

· ½ cup chia seeds

· 1 banana, mashed

· 1 cup almond milk (or cashew milk or any other milk alternative)

· 2 tablespoons maple syrup (or any other sweetener)

· ¼ cup walnuts, chopped

Directions:

1. In a medium bowl, combine the chia seeds, mashed banana, almond milk, and maple syrup. Mix until all ingredients are evenly incorporated.

2. Cover the bowl and place it in the refrigerator for at least 4 hours or overnight.

3. The next morning, remove the bowl from the fridge and stir in the chopped walnuts.

4. Serve with your favorite toppings and enjoy!

Cholesterol value per serving: Less than 10mg

Recipe 3: Almond Butter Blueberry Toast

Ingredients:

· 2 slices of whole wheat bread (or any other type of bread you prefer)

· 2 tablespoons almond butter

· ½ cup blueberries, fresh or frozen

· 1 teaspoon honey (optional)

Directions:

1. Toast the bread slices in a toaster or skillet over medium heat until golden brown and crispy.

2. Spread the almond butter evenly onto each slice of Toast.

3. Top with blueberries and drizzle with honey (optional).

4. Serve and enjoy!

Cholesterol value per serving: Less than 10mg

Recipe 4: Avocado Toast with Poached Egg

Ingredients:

· 2 slices of whole wheat bread (or any other type of bread you prefer)

· ½ avocado, mashed

· 1 egg, poached

· Salt and pepper to taste

· Chopped parsley (optional)

Directions:

1. Toast the bread slices in a toaster or skillet over medium heat until golden brown and crispy.

2. Spread the mashed avocado onto each slice of Toast.

3. Poach the egg (you can find instructions on how to do this online) and place it on top of one of the slices of Toast.

4. Sprinkle with salt and pepper to taste and chopped parsley (if desired).

5. Serve and enjoy!

Cholesterol value per serving: Less than 10mg

Recipe 5: Sweet Potato Toast with Avocado

Ingredients:

· 2 sweet potatoes, thinly sliced

· 1 avocado, mashed

· 2 tablespoons olive oil

· Salt and pepper to taste

· Chopped parsley (optional)

Directions:

1. Preheat the oven to 400°F.

2. Line a baking sheet with parchment paper and place the sliced sweet potatoes in a single layer. Drizzle with olive oil, salt, and pepper to taste.

3. Bake for 20 minutes or until the sweet potatoes are cooked.

4. Remove from the oven and spread the mashed avocado onto each slice of Toast.

5 Sprinkle with salt and pepper to taste and chopped parsley (if desired).

6. Serve and enjoy!

Cholesterol value per serving: Less than 10mg

RECIPE 6: Banana Oatmeal Pancakes

Ingredients:

· ½ cup rolled oats

· 1 banana, mashed

· ¼ teaspoon baking powder

· ¼ teaspoon ground cinnamon (optional)

· 2 tablespoons almond Milk (or any other milk alternative)

· 1 egg, lightly beaten

· 2 tablespoons coconut oil (or any other cooking oil of your choice)

Directions:

1. In a medium bowl, combine the oats, mashed banana, baking powder, and cinnamon (if using). Mix until all ingredients are evenly incorporated.

2. Pour in the almond milk and lightly beaten egg and stir until everything is well mixed.

3. Heat the coconut oil in a large skillet over medium

heat.

4. Once the oil is hot, spoon 1/4 cup of the batter onto the skillet for each pancake. Cook for 2-3 minutes or until the edges are golden brown and bubbles appear on the pancakes.

5. Flip the pancakes over and cook for 2-3 minutes or until cooked through.

6. Serve with your favorite toppings and enjoy!

Cholesterol value per serving: Less than 10mg

Recipe 7: Omelette with Spinach and Cherry Tomatoes

Ingredients:

· 2 eggs, lightly beaten
· ¼ cup spinach, chopped
· ½ cup cherry tomatoes, halved
· 1 tablespoon olive oil
· Salt and pepper to taste

Directions:

1. Mix the eggs with salt and pepper in a medium bowl. Mix until all ingredients are evenly incorporated.

2. Heat the olive oil in a large skillet over medium heat.

3. Once the oil is hot, add the spinach and cherry tomatoes to the skillet and cook for 2-3 minutes or until the vegetables are slightly softened.

4. Pour in the egg mixture and cook for 3-4 minutes or until cooked.

5. Serve and enjoy!

Cholesterol value per serving: Less than 10mg

Recipe 8: Zucchini Noodles with Avocado Pesto

Ingredients:

· 2 zucchinis, spiralized

· ½ avocado, mashed

· ¼ cup basil leaves, chopped

· 1 garlic clove, minced

· 2 tablespoons olive oil (or any other cooking oil of your choice)

· Salt and pepper to taste

Directions:

1. Combine the mashed avocado, basil, garlic, olive oil, and salt and pepper in a food processor. Process until smooth. Set aside.

2. Heat a large skillet over medium heat and add the spiralized zucchini noodles. Cook for 3-4 minutes or until slightly softened.

3. Mix in the avocado pesto until everything is well combined.

4. Serve and enjoy!

Cholesterol value per serving: Less than 10mg

RECIPE 9: Quinoa Bowl with Roasted Vegetables

Ingredients:

· 1 cup quinoa, cooked

· 1 bell pepper, chopped

· 2 cups broccoli florets

· 1 onion, chopped

· 2 tablespoons olive oil (or any other cooking oil of your choice)

· Salt and pepper to taste

Directions:

1. Preheat the oven to 400°F.

2. Toss the bell pepper, broccoli, onion with olive oil, salt, and pepper in a large bowl until everything is evenly coated.

3. Spread the vegetables onto a baking sheet lined with parchment paper and bake for 20 minutes or until cooked.

4. Place the quinoa in a large bowl and top it with the roasted vegetables. Mix until everything is well combined.

5. Serve and enjoy!

Cholesterol value per serving: Less than 10mg

RECIPE 10: Grilled Salmon with Mango Salsa

Ingredients:

· 2 salmon filets

· 1 mango, diced

· ½ red onion, diced

· 2 tablespoons lime juice

· 2 tablespoons olive oil (or any other cooking oil of your choice)

· Salt and pepper to taste

Directions:

1. Preheat the grill or a large skillet over medium heat.

2. Brush the salmon filets with olive oil, salt, and pepper, then place them on the grill or skillet. Cook for 4-5 minutes per side or until cooked through.

3. In a medium bowl, combine the mango, red onion, lime juice, and some salt and pepper. Mix until all ingredients are evenly incorporated.

4. Serve the grilled salmon with the mango salsa on top, and enjoy!

Cholesterol value per serving: Less than 10mg

Lunch Recipes

Recipe 1: Broccoli & Cheese Stuffed Portobello Mushrooms

Ingredients:

· 4 portobello mushrooms caps, stems removed
· 1 teaspoon olive oil
· 2 cups broccoli florets, chopped finely
· ½ cup onion, diced
· ¼ teaspoon garlic powder
· ½ cup shredded cheese (of your choice)
· Salt and pepper to taste

Directions:

1. Preheat the oven to 375°F.

2. Heat a large skillet over medium heat and add the olive oil. Once the oil is hot, add the broccoli, onion, garlic powder, salt and pepper. Cook for 5-7 minutes or until the vegetables are tender.

3. Place the mushroom caps on a baking sheet lined with parchment paper and gill side up.

4. Spoon the broccoli mixture onto each mushroom cap and top them with shredded cheese. Bake for 10 minutes or until the cheese is melted and golden brown.

5. Serve and enjoy!

Cholesterol value per serving: Less than 10mg

RECIPE 2: Eggplant Lasagna Rolls

Ingredients:

· 1 eggplant, sliced lengthwise into 8 slices
· ¼ cup ricotta cheese (or any other type of cheese of your choice)
· ½ cup spinach, chopped

· 2 tablespoons olive oil (or any other cooking oil of your choice)

· ¼ cup marinara sauce

· Salt and pepper to taste

Directions:

1. Preheat the oven to 375°F.

2. Heat a large skillet over medium heat and add the olive oil. Once the oil is hot, add the eggplant slices and cook for 3-4 minutes per side or until lightly browned.

3. In a small bowl, combine the ricotta cheese with the spinach, salt and pepper. Mix until all ingredients are evenly incorporated.

4. Spread a spoonful of marinara sauce onto each eggplant slice and top it with some of the ricotta cheese mixture. Roll each slice up and place them onto a baking sheet lined with parchment paper.

5. Bake for 15 minutes or until the eggplant rolls are heated.

6. Serve and enjoy!

Cholesterol value per serving: Less than 10mg

RECIPE 3: Lentil Stew with Sweet Potatoes

Ingredients:

· 1 cup red lentils, rinsed and drained

· 2 sweet potatoes, peeled and cubed

· 4 cups vegetable broth (or any other type of broth of your choice)

· 1 onion, diced

· 2 garlic cloves, minced

· 1 teaspoon paprika powder

· 2 tablespoons olive oil (or any other cooking oil of your choice)

· Salt and pepper to taste

Directions:

1. Heat the olive oil in a large pot over medium heat. Once the oil is hot, add the onion and garlic and cook for 3 minutes or until softened.

2. Add the sweet potatoes, lentils, vegetable broth, paprika powder, salt, and pepper to the pot and bring it to a boil.

3. Reduce the heat to low and simmer for 20 minutes or until the lentils are tender.

4. Serve and enjoy!

Cholesterol value per serving: Less than 10mg

RECIPE 4: Spinach & Feta Quiche

Ingredients:

· 8 eggs

· 2 cups spinach, chopped

· ½ cup feta cheese, crumbled

· ¼ cup sun-dried tomatoes, chopped

· 1 onion, diced

· 2 tablespoons olive oil (or any other cooking oil of your choice)

· Salt and pepper to taste

Directions:

1. Preheat the oven to 375°F.

2. Heat a large skillet over medium heat and add the olive oil. Once the oil is hot, add the onion and cook for 3 minutes or until softened. Add the spinach and sun-dried tomatoes and cook for another 2-3 minutes or until the spinach has wilted.

3. Beat the eggs in a large bowl and season with salt and

pepper to taste. Add the feta cheese and spinach mixture until everything is well combined.

4. Pour the egg mixture into a greased 9-inch pie dish and bake for 30 minutes or until the top is golden brown.

5. Serve and enjoy!

Cholesterol value per serving: Less than 10mg

RECIPE 5: Baked Falafel with Cucumber & Tomato Salad

Ingredients:

· 1 can chickpeas, rinsed and drained

· ½ cup fresh parsley, chopped

· 4 garlic cloves, minced

· 1 teaspoon cumin powder

· 2 tablespoons olive oil (or any other cooking oil of your choice)

· 1 cucumber, diced

· 2 tomatoes, diced

· Juice from 1 lemon

· Salt and pepper to taste

Directions:

1. Preheat the oven to 375°F.

2. Place the chickpeas, parsley, garlic, and cumin into a food processor and blend until everything is well combined. Add salt and pepper to taste.

3. Use your hands to form little balls from the chickpea mixture and place them onto a baking sheet lined with parchment paper. Brush the falafel balls with olive oil and bake for 15 minutes or until golden brown.

4. In a medium bowl, combine the cucumbers, tomatoes, lemon juice, salt and pepper. Mix until all ingredients are evenly incorporated.

5. Serve the falafel balls with the cucumber salad, and enjoy!

Cholesterol value per serving: Less than 10mg

Recipe 6: Vegetable Fried Rice with Tofu

Ingredients:

· 1 block of extra firm tofu, cubed

· 2 cups cooked rice (of your choice)

· 1 cup broccoli florets, chopped finely

· ½ cup carrots, diced

· 2 tablespoons olive oil (or any other cooking oil of your choice)

· 2 tablespoons soy sauce

· 1 teaspoon sesame oil

· Salt and pepper to taste

Directions:

1. Heat a large skillet over medium heat and add the olive oil. Once the oil is hot, add the tofu cubes and cook for 3-4 minutes per side or until golden brown.

2. Add the broccoli, carrots, cooked rice, soy sauce, sesame oil, salt, and pepper to the skillet and cook for 5 minutes or until all ingredients are heated.

3. Serve and enjoy!

Cholesterol value per serving: Less than 10mg

Recipe 7: Eggplant Parmesan

Ingredients:

· 1 eggplant, sliced into 8 slices

· ½ cup marinara sauce

· ¼ cup parmesan cheese, grated

· 2 tablespoons olive oil (or any other cooking oil of your choice)

· Salt and pepper to taste

Directions:

1. Preheat the oven to 375°F.

2. Heat a large skillet over medium heat and add the olive oil. Once the oil is hot, add the eggplant slices and cook for 3-4 minutes per side or until lightly browned.

3. Spread some marinara sauce onto each eggplant slice and top it with some of the parmesan cheese.

4. Bake for 15 minutes or until the eggplant slices are heated through, and the cheese is melted and golden brown.

5. Serve and enjoy!

Cholesterol value per serving: Less than 10mg

RECIPE 8: Lentil Burgers with Spinach & Avocado

Ingredients:

· 1 cup dry lentils, rinsed and drained

· 1 onion, diced

· 2 garlic cloves, minced

· ½ cup cooked brown rice

· 1 teaspoon cumin powder

· 2 tablespoons olive oil (or any other cooking oil of your choice)

· 1 avocado, sliced

· 2 cups spinach, chopped

· Salt and pepper to taste

Directions:

1. Heat a large skillet over medium heat and add the olive oil. Once the oil is hot, add the onion and garlic and cook for 3 minutes or until softened. Add the lentils, brown

rice, cumin powder, salt, and pepper to the skillet and cook for 5 minutes or until everything is heated.

2. Remove the mixture from the heat and let it cool slightly before adding it to a bowl. Use a fork or potato masher to mash the lentil mixture until it becomes a paste-like consistency.

3. Form 9 patties with your hands from the lentil mixture and place them onto a baking sheet lined with parchment paper.

4. Bake for 20 minutes until the patties are golden brown and crispy.

5. Serve each burger topped with spinach and avocado slices, and enjoy!

Cholesterol value per serving: Less than 10mg

RECIPE 9: Roasted Vegetable & Tofu Stir Fry

Ingredients:

· 1 block of extra firm tofu, cubed

· 2 cups broccoli florets

· ½ cup carrots, diced

· 2 tablespoons olive oil (or any other cooking oil of your choice)

· 3 garlic cloves, minced

· 2 tablespoons soy sauce

· 1 teaspoon sesame oil

· Salt and pepper to taste

Directions:

1. Preheat the oven to 375°F.

2. Place the broccoli and carrots onto a baking sheet lined with parchment paper and drizzle them with olive oil, salt, and pepper. Roast for 20 minutes or until the vegetables are tender.

3. Heat a large skillet over medium heat and add the olive oil. Once the oil is hot, add the tofu cubes and cook for 3-4 minutes per side or until golden brown.

4. Add the roasted broccoli and carrots to the skillet with garlic, soy sauce, sesame oil, and salt and pepper to taste. Cook for 5 minutes or until everything is heated through.

5. Serve and enjoy!

Cholesterol value per serving: Less than 10mg

Recipe 10: Grilled Eggplant & Zucchini with Feta Cheese

Ingredients:

· 1 eggplant, sliced into 8 slices

· 2 zucchinis, sliced into 8 slices

· ¼ cup feta cheese, crumbled

· 2 tablespoons olive oil (or any other cooking oil of your choice)

· Salt and pepper to taste

Directions:

1. Heat a grill pan over medium heat and brush with olive oil. Once the pan is hot, add the eggplant and zucchini slices and cook for 3-4 minutes per side or until lightly browned.

2. Sprinkle each slice with feta cheese and cook for 1 more minute or until the cheese is melted.

3. Serve and enjoy!

Cholesterol value per serving: Less than 10mg

Dinner Recipes

Recipe 1: Grilled Salmon with Roasted Vegetables

Ingredients:

· 4 salmon fillets (4-6 ounces each)

· 2 cups broccoli florets

· ½ cup carrots, diced

· 2 tablespoons olive oil (or any other cooking oil of your choice)

· Salt and pepper to taste

Directions:

1. Preheat the oven to 375°F.

2. Place the broccoli and carrots onto a baking sheet lined with parchment paper and drizzle them with olive oil, salt, and pepper. Roast for 20 minutes or until the vegetables are tender.

3. Heat a grill pan over medium heat and brush with olive oil. Once the pan is hot, add the salmon fillets and cook for 4-5 minutes per side or until cooked through (test with a fork).

4. Serve each salmon fillet topped with roasted vegetables, and enjoy!

Cholesterol value per serving: Less than 10mg

RECIPE 2: Zucchini & Mushroom Lasagna

Ingredients:

· 1 large zucchini, sliced into long strips

· 8 ounces mushrooms, diced

· 2 tablespoons olive oil (or any other cooking oil of your choice)

· ½ cup marinara sauce

· ¼ cup parmesan cheese, grated

· Salt and pepper to taste

Directions:

1. Preheat the oven to 375°F.

2. Heat a large skillet over medium heat and add the olive oil. Once the oil is hot, add the mushrooms and cook

for 3-4 minutes or until softened. Add some salt and pepper to taste.

3. Spread some marinara sauce onto the bottom of a baking dish and layer it with half of the zucchini strips, mushroom mixture, and parmesan cheese. Repeat the layers one more time.

4. Bake for 25 minutes or until the zucchini is tender and the cheese is melted and golden brown.

5. Serve and enjoy!

Cholesterol value per serving: Less than 10mg

RECIPE 3: Baked Sweet Potato Fries with Chipotle Ranch Dip

Ingredients:

· 4 large sweet potatoes, cut into thin wedges

· 2 tablespoons olive oil (or any other cooking oil of your choice)

· ¼ cup plain Greek yogurt

· 2 tablespoons chipotle peppers in adobo sauce, diced

· 1 tablespoon lime juice

· Salt and pepper to taste

Directions:

1. Preheat the oven to 375°F.

2. Place the sweet potato wedges onto a baking sheet lined with parchment paper and drizzle them with olive oil, salt, and pepper. Bake for 25 minutes or until the fries are golden brown and crispy.

3. Meanwhile, in a small bowl, mix the Greek yogurt, chipotle peppers, and lime juice. Season with salt and pepper to taste.

4. Serve the sweet potato fries hot with the chipotle ranch dip, and enjoy!

Cholesterol value per serving: Less than 10mg

RECIPE 4: Grilled Portobello Mushrooms with Quinoa Salad

Ingredients:

· 4 portobello mushrooms, stems removed

· 2 tablespoons olive oil (or any other cooking oil of your choice)

· 2 cups cooked quinoa

· ½ cup corn kernels

· 1 avocado, diced

· 2 tablespoons lime juice

· Salt and pepper to taste

Directions:

1. Heat a grill pan over medium heat and brush with some olive oil. Once the pan is hot, add the portobello mushrooms and cook for 5 minutes per side or until tender.

2. In a large bowl, mix the cooked quinoa, corn kernels, avocado, lime juice, and salt and pepper to taste.

3. Serve each portobello mushroom topped with some quinoa salad, and enjoy!

Cholesterol value per serving: Less than 10mg

RECIPE 5: Stuffed Bell Peppers with Quinoa & Feta Cheese

Ingredients:

· 4 bell peppers, tops removed and seeded

· 2 cups cooked quinoa

· ½ cup feta cheese, crumbled

· 2 tablespoons olive oil (or any other cooking oil of your choice)

· ½ teaspoon garlic powder

· Salt and pepper to taste

Directions:

1. Preheat the oven to 375°F.

2. Place the bell peppers onto a baking sheet lined with parchment paper and drizzle them with olive oil, salt, and pepper. Bake for 15 minutes or until tender.

3. Meanwhile, in a large bowl, mix the cooked quinoa, feta cheese, garlic powder, and salt and pepper to taste.

4. Fill each bell pepper with some of the quinoa mixture and bake for 15 more minutes or until the cheese is melted and golden brown.

5. Serve and enjoy!

Cholesterol value per serving: Less than 10mg

Recipe 6: Roasted Cauliflower & Chickpeas with Shallot Vinaigrette

Ingredients:

· 4 cups cauliflower florets

· 1 can chickpeas, drained and rinsed

· 2 tablespoons olive oil (or any other cooking oil of your choice)

· 1 shallot, finely chopped

· 2 tablespoons balsamic vinegar

· Salt and pepper to taste

Directions:

1. Preheat the oven to 375°F.

2. Place the cauliflower florets onto a baking sheet lined with parchment paper and drizzle them with olive oil, salt, and pepper. Roast for 20 minutes or until tender.

3. Meanwhile, in a small bowl, mix the shallot, balsamic vinegar, and salt and pepper to taste.

4. Once the cauliflower is cooked, add the chickpeas to the baking sheet and toss with some vinaigrette. Bake for 10 more minutes or until the chickpeas are crispy.

5. Serve and enjoy!

Cholesterol value per serving: Less than 10mg

RECIPE 7: Baked Sweet Potato & Egg Hash

Ingredients:

· 2 large sweet potatoes, cubed

· 4 eggs

· 2 tablespoons olive oil (or any other cooking oil of your choice)

· Salt and pepper to taste

Directions:

1. Preheat the oven to 375°F.

2. Place the sweet potatoes onto a baking sheet lined with parchment paper and drizzle them with olive oil, salt, and pepper. Roast for 25 minutes or until tender.

3. Once the sweet potatoes are cooked, create 4 wells in the baking sheet and crack an egg into each one. Bake for 8-10 more minutes or until the eggs are cooked to your preference.

4. Serve and enjoy!

Cholesterol value per serving: Less than 10mg

RECIPE 8: Sweet Potato & Black Bean Quesadillas

Ingredients:

· 2 large sweet potatoes, cubed

· 1 can black beans, drained and rinsed

· 4 whole wheat wraps

· ½ cup cheddar cheese, grated

· 2 tablespoons olive oil (or any other cooking oil of your choice)

· Salt and pepper to taste

Directions:

1. Preheat the oven to 375°F.

2. Place the sweet potatoes onto a baking sheet lined with parchment paper and drizzle them with olive oil, salt, and pepper. Roast for 25 minutes or until tender.

3. Meanwhile, in a medium bowl, mash the black beans with a fork.

4. Divide the mashed beans and roasted sweet potatoes between the whole wheat wraps and top them with cheddar cheese. Fold each wrap into a quesadilla shape and press lightly to seal them shut.

5. Place the quesadillas onto a baking sheet lined with parchment paper and bake for 8-10 minutes or until the cheese is melted and golden brown.

6. Serve and enjoy!

Cholesterol value per serving: Less than 10mg

RECIPE 9: Baked Banana Bread with Walnuts

Ingredients:

· 2 cups all-purpose flour

· ½ teaspoon baking soda

· ¼ teaspoon salt

· 1 cup packed brown sugar

· 3 ripe bananas, mashed

· ⅓ cup olive oil (or any other cooking oil of your choice)

· 1 teaspoon vanilla extract

· 2 large eggs, lightly beaten

· ½ cup walnuts, chopped

Directions:

1. Preheat the oven to 350°F. Grease a 9x5 inch loaf pan and set aside.

2. In a large bowl, whisk together the flour, baking soda, and salt.

3. In a medium bowl, mix the brown sugar, mashed bananas, olive oil, vanilla extract, and eggs until well combined. Pour the wet ingredients into the dry ingredients and stir until just combined. Do not overmix!

4. Gently fold the chopped walnuts and pour the batter into the prepared loaf pan. Bake for 40-45 minutes or until a toothpick inserted into the center of the loaf comes out clean.

5. Let the banana bread cool in the pan for 10 minutes before transferring it onto a cooling rack to cool completely.

6. Serve and enjoy!

Cholesterol value per serving: Less than 10mg

RECIPE 10: Lentil & Zucchini Fritters

Ingredients:

· 2 cups cooked lentils

· 2 zucchinis, grated

· 1 onion, finely chopped

· 2 tablespoons olive oil (or any other cooking oil of your choice)

· ½ teaspoon garlic powder

· Salt and pepper to taste

Directions:

1. In a large bowl, mix the cooked lentils, grated zucchini, onion, garlic powder, and salt and pepper to taste.

2. Form 10-12 fritters with your hands and place them onto a plate lined with parchment or waxed paper. Refrigerate for 15-20 minutes or until they become firm.

3. Heat the olive oil in a large skillet over medium heat and place the fritters into it. Cook for 5-7 minutes per side or until golden brown and crispy.

4. Serve and enjoy!

Cholesterol value per serving: Less than 10mg

Snacks and Desserts

Recipe 1: Carrot Cake Oatmeal Cookies

Ingredients:

· 2 cups rolled oats

· 1 cup grated carrots

· ½ cup chopped walnuts

· ½ teaspoon baking powder

· ¼ teaspoon ground cinnamon

· 2 tablespoons olive oil (or any other cooking oil of your choice)

· 3 tablespoons pure maple syrup

· 2 tablespoons almond butter

Directions:

1. Preheat the oven to 375°F. Line a baking sheet with parchment paper and set aside.

2. In a large bowl, mix the oats, grated carrots, walnuts, baking powder, and cinnamon until well combined.

3. In a small bowl, mix the olive oil, maple syrup, and almond butter until well combined. Pour the wet ingredients into the dry ingredients and stir until just combined. Do not overmix!

4. Scoop about 1 tablespoon of the cookie dough onto the prepared baking sheet and use your hand to flatten them slightly. Bake for 10-12 minutes or until the edges of the cookies are golden brown.

5. Let the cookies cool in the pan for 10 minutes before transferring them onto a cooling rack to cool completely.

6. Serve and enjoy!

Cholesterol value per serving: Less than 10mg

RECIPE 2: Coconut & Pomegranate Chia Pudding

Ingredients:

· 2 cups unsweetened almond milk

· ½ cup chia seeds

· ¼ cup shredded coconut, plus more for topping

· ¼ cup pomegranate arils (or any other type of fruit of your choice)

· 2 tablespoons pure maple syrup (or any other sweetener of your choice)

· 1 teaspoon vanilla extract

Directions:

1. In a medium bowl, mix the almond milk, chia seeds, shredded coconut, pomegranate arils, maple syrup, and vanilla extract until well combined. Cover the bowl with plastic wrap and refrigerate for at least 2 hours or overnight.

2. Serve the chia pudding with shredded coconut and pomegranate arils.

3. Enjoy!

Cholesterol value per serving: Less than 10mg

RECIPE 3: Peanut Butter & Jelly Energy Bites

Ingredients:

· 1 cup rolled oats

· ½ cup peanut butter (or any other nut or seed butter of your choice)

· ½ cup dried cranberries

· ¼ cup pure maple syrup (or any other sweetener of your choice)

· 2 tablespoons chia seeds

· 2 tablespoons almond flour

· 1 teaspoon vanilla extract

· Pinch of salt

Directions:

1. In a medium bowl, mix the rolled oats, peanut butter, dried cranberries, maple syrup, chia seeds, almond flour, vanilla extract, and salt until well combined.

2. Form 10-12 energy bites with your hands and place them onto a plate lined with parchment or waxed paper. Refrigerate for 1 hour or until they become firm.

3. Serve and enjoy!

Cholesterol value per serving: Less than 10mg

RECIPE 4: Chocolate Peanut Butter Banana Smoothie Bowl

Ingredients:

· 2 frozen bananas, sliced

· ½ cup creamy peanut butter

· ¼ cup cocoa powder

· 1 tablespoon pure maple syrup (or any other sweetener of your choice)

· ¼ teaspoon ground cinnamon

· ¾ cup unsweetened almond milk (or any other liquid of your choice)

· Toppings: granola, nuts, seeds, or any other topping of your choice

Directions:

1. In a blender or food processor, combine the frozen

bananas, peanut butter, cocoa powder, maple syrup, cinnamon, and almond milk until smooth and creamy.

2. Pour the smoothie into a bowl and top with granola, nuts, seeds, or any other toppings you choose.

3. Serve and enjoy!

Cholesterol value per serving: Less than 10mg

RECIPE 5: Banana Coconut Muffins

Ingredients:

· 2 cups all-purpose flour
· ½ cup sugar
· 1 teaspoon baking powder
· ¼ teaspoon baking soda
· ¼ teaspoon salt
· 3 large ripe bananas, mashed
· ½ cup coconut oil (or any other cooking oil of your choice)
· ¼ cup coconut yogurt (or any other type of yogurt of your choice)
· 2 teaspoons pure vanilla extract
· ½ cup shredded coconut, plus more for topping

Directions:

1. Preheat the oven to 375°F. Grease a muffin tin with some oil and set aside.

2. In a medium bowl, mix the flour, sugar, baking powder, baking soda, and salt until well combined.

3. In a small bowl, mix the mashed bananas, coconut oil, coconut yogurt, and vanilla extract until well combined. Pour the wet ingredients into the dry ingredients and stir until just combined. Do not overmix!

4. Divide the batter among the muffin cups and sprinkle with shredded coconut. Bake for 20-25 minutes or until a

toothpick inserted into the center of a muffin comes out clean.

5. Let the muffins cool in the pan for 10 minutes before transferring them onto a cooling rack to cool completely.

6. Serve and enjoy!

Recipe 6: Chocolate Coconut Macaroons

Ingredients:

· 2 cups shredded coconut

· 1/3 cup cocoa powder

· ⅓ cup pure maple syrup (or any other sweetener of your choice)

· 2 tablespoons coconut oil (or any other cooking oil of your choice)

· ¼ teaspoon salt

· 1 teaspoon pure vanilla extract

· Toppings: chocolate chips, nuts, seeds, or any other topping of your choice

Directions:

1. Preheat the oven to 350°F. Line a baking sheet with parchment paper and set aside.

2. In a medium bowl, mix the shredded coconut, cocoa powder, maple syrup, coconut oil, salt, and vanilla extract until well combined.

3. Form about 16-18 macaroons with your hands and place them onto the prepared baking sheet. Sprinkle some chocolate chips, nuts, and seeds over each macaroon (or any other topping you choose).

4. Bake for 12-15 minutes or until the edges of the macaroons are golden brown.

5. Let the macaroons cool on the pan for 10 minutes

before transferring them onto a cooling rack to cool completely.

6. Serve and enjoy!

Cholesterol value per serving: Less than 10mg

RECIPE 7: Overnight Raspberry Chia Pudding

Ingredients:

· 2 cups unsweetened almond milk

· ½ cup chia seeds

· ¼ cup fresh raspberries (or any other type of fruit of your choice)

· 2 tablespoons pure maple syrup (or any other sweetener of your choice)

· 1 teaspoon vanilla extract

· Toppings: granola, nuts, seeds, or any other topping of your choice

Directions:

1. In a medium bowl, mix the almond milk, chia seeds, raspberries, maple syrup, and vanilla extract until well combined. Cover the bowl with plastic wrap and refrigerate for at least 8 hours or overnight.

2. Serve the chia pudding with fresh raspberries and your favorite topping.

3. Enjoy!

Cholesterol value per serving: Less than 10mg

RECIPE 8: Peanut Butter & Jelly Overnight Oats

Ingredients:

· 1 cup rolled oats

· ½ cup creamy peanut butter (or any other nut or seed butter of your choice)

· ¼ cup dried cranberries

· 2 tablespoons chia seeds

· 1 teaspoon vanilla extract

· Pinch of salt

· ¾ cup unsweetened almond milk (or any other liquid of your choice)

· 2 tablespoons pure maple syrup (or any other sweetener of your choice)

· Toppings: fresh fruit, nuts, and seeds, or any other topping of your choice

Directions:

1. In a medium bowl, mix the rolled oats, peanut butter, dried cranberries, chia seeds, vanilla extract, and salt until well combined.

2. Add the almond milk, maple syrup, and any other topping of choice and stir until everything is evenly distributed.

3. Cover the bowl with plastic wrap and refrigerate overnight or for at least 8 hours.

4. Serve the oatmeal with fresh fruit, nuts, seeds, or any other topping you choose.

5. Enjoy!

Cholesterol value per serving: Less than 10mg

Recipe 9: Crunchy Trail Mix

Ingredients:

· 1 cup rolled oats

· ½ cup roasted almonds

· ¼ cup dried cranberries

· ¼ cup dark chocolate chips

· 2 tablespoons chia seeds

· 2 tablespoons sesame seeds

· Pinch of salt

Directions:

1. In a large bowl, mix the rolled oats, almonds, dried cranberries, dark chocolate chips, chia seeds, sesame seeds, and salt until well combined.

2. Divide the mixture into small baggies or store in an airtight container for individual servings.

3. Serve and enjoy!

Cholesterol value per serving: Less than 10mg

RECIPE 10: No-Bake Peanut Butter Energy Bites

Ingredients:

· 2 cups rolled oats

· 1 cup creamy peanut butter (or any other nut or seed butter of your choice)

· ½ cup honey (or any other sweetener of your choice)

· ¼ cup sesame seeds

· ¼ cup chia seeds

· Toppings: chocolate chips, coconut flakes, or any other topping of your choice

Directions:

1. In a medium bowl, mix the rolled oats, peanut butter, honey, sesame seeds, and chia seeds until well combined.

2. Form about 16-18 balls with your hands and roll them in the desired topping.

3. Place the energy bites on a parchment paper-covered baking sheet and refrigerate for at least 1 hour before serving.

4. Serve and enjoy!

Cholesterol value per serving: Less than 10mg

5

BEYOND DIET: ADDITIONAL
LIFESTYLE CONSIDERATIONS

The role of physical activity in cholesterol management

Physical activity regularly is crucial to maintaining healthy cholesterol levels. Exercise helps to burn excess calories and can assist with bringing down your LDL ("terrible") cholesterol levels while raising your HDL ("good") cholesterol levels.

According to the American Heart Association, adults are encouraged to aim for at least 30 minutes of moderate-force active work five days a week, including walking, jogging, or swimming. It is also important to include strength-training exercises twice weekly for overall health and wellness.

Regarding physical activity, it is important not to overdo it! Aiming for too much exercise can be detrimental as it can increase the risk of injury and exhaustion. Additionally, it is important to warm up before exercise and cool down afterward.

It will help to reduce the risk of injury and allow your body to ease into activity before gradually building up intensity levels.

Finally, remember rest days! It is important to give your body time to recover from physical activity as this allows for optimal performance during future workouts and helps to promote overall health. Remember – when it comes to physical activity, quality over quantity is key! Take small but consistent steps toward a healthy lifestyle, and you will be well on your way toward improved cholesterol management.

STRESS REDUCTION TECHNIQUES for overall cardiovascular health

Stress can harm physical and mental health, with research linking high-stress levels to increased risk of heart disease. It is important to be mindful of the body's response to stress and practice techniques that can help manage it healthily.

Here are some tips for reducing stress:

• Listen to relaxing music or find another entertainment that helps you unwind, such as reading or watching a movie.
• Get moving! Practice is a magnificent type of pressure help – try activities such as yoga, tai chi, walking, or dancing that don't involve competition or pressure.
• Take short breaks throughout the day and allow yourself time to relax.

• Spend some time outdoors – walk in the park, hike, or sit and enjoy nature's beauty.

• Practice mindfulness and meditation techniques to help clear your mind and focus on the present moment.

• Connect with others – talk to family, friends or even join a support group for extra support if needed.

• Unplug from technology occasionally – find activities like painting, cooking, or gardening that don't involve screens!

REMEMBER: reducing stress is ultimately about finding what works best for you as an individual. Try different strategies until you find something that clicks; make it part of your daily routine to maintain a healthy stress level and overall cardiovascular health.

SMOKING cessation and its impact on cholesterol levels

Smoking can majorly impact cholesterol levels, as damage to blood vessel walls makes them more susceptible to damage from fatty deposits. In addition, cigarette smoke contains toxins and other harmful compounds that increase LDL ("terrible") cholesterol levels and reduce HDL ("good") cholesterol levels.

Quitting smoking is an important step towards improving your overall health – you will reap the benefits of improved cardiovascular health and lower your risk of stroke and cancer.

· · ·

HERE ARE **some tips for quitting:**

• Set a quit date – make sure it is realistic, and don't beat yourself up if you slip up or need to reset the date.

• Tell your friends and family about your decision – having support from the people around you can make a big difference.

• Throw away cigarettes and lighters to remove temptations as much as possible.

• Find healthier activities to replace smoking – try going for walks, yoga, or painting to help distract you from cravings.

• Avoid places and situations that trigger cravings – if you typically smoke after meals, try taking a post-meal walk instead.

• Consider nicotine replacement therapy (NRT) products such as patches, gum, or lozenges under the guidance of a healthcare professional.

• Don't give up! Quitting can be difficult, but it is worth the effort – the benefits to your health will be well worth it.

Stopping smoking can affect cholesterol levels, so consider these tips and quit today!

THE IMPORTANCE **of regular health check-ups and medication compliance**

Regular health check-ups are essential to maintaining good health, as they allow your doctor to monitor changes in your body's condition over time.

By getting regular check-ups, you can take proactive steps to address any potential problems and reduce the possibility of contracting a more severe disease or medical condition.

Regarding cholesterol management, regular check-ups are important for monitoring your cholesterol levels so that you can work with your doctor to make necessary lifestyle and dietary changes. Additionally, suppose you have been prescribed medication for high cholesterol. In that case, it is important to be consistent with taking them as directed – this will ensure the optimal effectiveness of the medication and help keep cholesterol levels within the desired range.

Finally, remember that health check-ups should be tailored to your needs. Depending on your age, gender, and family history, you may need more or less frequent visits – talk to your doctor about what makes the most sense for you.

Regular health check-ups and medication compliance are key components of successful cholesterol management. Work with your doctor to develop an individualized plan so that you can stay informed about any changes in your body's condition and make necessary lifestyle adjustments when needed. It will help ensure a long and healthy life!

CONCLUSIOIN

"The Complete Guide to Cholesterol: Low Cholesterol Foods and High Cholesterol Foods to Avoid" empowers you with knowledge and practical tools to make informed choices about your diet. By incorporating low-cholesterol foods and limiting high-cholesterol foods, you can take proactive steps toward managing cholesterol levels and promoting heart health. Consulting with healthcare professionals or registered dietitians is crucial for personalized advice based on your unique health circumstances. With this book as your guide, embark on a journey toward a heart-healthy lifestyle and better overall well-being.

Made in the USA
Monee, IL
16 November 2023